Practical
Forensic Medicine

Practical
Forensic Medicine

K Thangaraj MD

Professor and Head
Department of Forensic Medicine
SRM Medical College and Research Centre
Potheri, Kattankulathur, Tamil Nadu 603 203

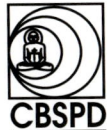

CBS **Publishers & Distributors** Pvt Ltd

New Delhi • Bengaluru • Chennai • Kochi • Kolkata • Lucknow • Mumbai
Hyderabad • Jharkhand • Nagpur • Patna • Pune • Uttarakhand

Practical
Forensic Medicine

ISBN: 978-81-239-2834-0

Copyright © Author and Publisher

First Edition: 2016

Reprint: 2021, 2024

Published by Satish Kumar Jain and Produced by Varun Jain for

CBS Publishers & Distributors Pvt Ltd

4819/XI Prahlad Street, 24 Ansari Road, Daryaganj, New Delhi 110 002, India
Ph: 011-23289259, 23266838   Website: www.cbspd.com
                                                              e-mail: delhi@cbspd.com
Corporate Office: 204 FIE, Industrial Area, Patparganj, Delhi 110 092
Ph: 011-4934 4934   Fax: 011-4934 4935   e-mail: publishing@cbspd.com; publicity@cbspd.com

Branches

- **Bengaluru:** Seema House 2975, 17th Cross, K.R. Road, Banasankari 2nd Stage, Bengaluru 560 070, Karnataka, India
  Ph: +91-80-26771678/79   Fax: +91-80-26771680   e-mail: bangalore@cbspd.com
- **Chennai:** 7, Subbaraya Street, Shenoy Nagar, Chennai 600 030, Tamil Nadu, India
  Ph: +91-44-26680620, 26681266   Fax: +91-44-42032115   e-mail: chennai@cbspd.com
- **Kochi:** 42/1325, 1326, Power House Road, Opp KSEB, Power House, Ernakulam 682 018, Kerala, India
  Ph: +91-484-4059061-65   Fax: +91-484-4059065   e-mail: kochi@cbspd.com
- **Kolkata:** 147, Hind Ceramics Compound, 1st Floor, Nilgunj Road, Belghoria, Kolkata-700056
  West Bengal, India
  Ph: 033-25633055, 033-25633056   e-mail: kolkata@cbspd.com
- **Lucknow:** Basement, Khushnuma Complex, 7-Meerabai Marg (Behind Jawahar Bhawan), Lucknow 226001, India
  Ph: 0522-4000032   e-mail: tiwari.lucknow@cbspd.com
- **Mumbai:** PWD Shed. Gala no. 25/26, Ramchandra Bhatt Marg, Next to JJ Hospital Gate no. 2, Opp. Union Bank of India Noorbaug
  Mumbai-400009, Maharashtra, India
  Ph: 022-66661880/89   e-mail: mumbai@cbspd.com

Representatives

- **Hyderabad** 0-9885175004   • **Jharkhand** 0-9811541605   • **Nagpur**   0-8692091830
- **Patna**   0-9334159340   • **Pune**   0-9664372571   • **Uttarakhand** 0-9716462459

Printed at HT Media Ltd, Greater Noida, UP, India

Foreword

Forensic medicine is one of the most fascinating and intriguing areas of study in the medical field. The rich experience gained during the forensic examinations of a diverse range of cases goes a long way in shaping the expertise of forensic pathologists. This concise, student-friendly practical book is a valuable text to update the skills during the course of study and even afterwards. Practical examination is vital in this field of study, as throughout one's service, there are opportunities to examine clinical forensic medicine cases. When the singular art of examination has been mastered at the undergraduate level with this book, the medical officer would definitely reap a worthwhile harvest with the knowledge gleaned from this remarkable presentation. Medical students are definitely at a constructive advantage that can only be dreamed of, as this book includes the entire set of exercises necessary for a thorough preparation and performance at the undergraduate practical examination. This book offers a complete array of study material, namely self-explanatory photographs, charts, tables, medicolegal certificates, description of spotters, evaluation questions and answers, along with the relevant section of the Indian Penal Code at the end of each chapter. These materials have considerably eased the preparatory work for the examination. This challenging subject of forensic medicine and toxicology has been admiringly encapsulated in this succinct, comprehensive and clear practical text.

With a surge in crime, particularly rape and age cases and suspicious cases presenting themselves daily, this book is also a useful resource for medical officers. With the steady progress of technological advances to deal with a plethora of crimes, the fundamental examination of the victim/accused in a crime always occupies the basis of any medicolegal examination. Time and again, medical officers are taken by surprise when the defence attorney needs a clarification or an explanation of a medicolegal term or a case. This is a useful book to refer to, before taking the stand in the witness box.

I am delighted to have read this book and the learned author has made the subject interesting and easy to understand. I would definitely recommend this book to all medical officers in the Casualty Department who examine wounds and drunkenness cases daily. Furthermore, all government hospitals must have a copy of this book to assist the doctors in issuing medicolegal certificates. Additionally, public prosecutors should have this book to adequately prepare their cases. This book is a necessary resource at police stations to assist police officers in preparing and recording the 161 [2] statement. Medical officers in gynaecology departments should read the chapters "Sexual Offence—Examination" and "Age Estimation" before issuing their certificates. They should all remember that *justice delayed is justice denied*, and I sincerely hope that this book would assist in the timely dispatch of all medicolegal certificates.

Dr Cecilia Cyril
Former Director
Institute of Forensic Medicine
Madras Medical College, Chennai

Preface

Forensic medicine is an applied science of medicine encompassing the knowledge of all the branches of medical fraternity. In present days almost all offences against the human body require a medical opinion in order to deliver an impeccable and impartial justice in law courts; hence a basic knowledge of forensic medicine is mandatory to every doctor to confirm with the needs of law. The primary interest of forensic medicine is to provide the source of information about forensic aspects of medical science and the other related fields in turn to give a sound service to the medical officers, investigative agency and law enforcing authorities.

This book has been designed to train the medical student to interpret knowledge of medical science bearing in mind the statutory laws, in order to render service to the legal fraternity to insure justice to the needed. Practical work in forensic medicine is nothing but observation of facts, collection of evidences, construction of right inferences based on medicolegal examination of the living or dead body since there is no place for vagueness or ambiguity in offering medical opinion.

Forensic medicine continues to advance with scientific techniques and laboratory investigations to support and enhance the administration of criminal justice and impartial dispensation of justice. Hope this book will assist and reinforce all the necessary academic forensic requirements.

I sincerely thank my family members, friends, colleagues and well wishers for their encouragement in preparing this book. I specially thank Dr V Chitra for her encouragement and typographical work.

K Thangaraj

Contents

Introduction

Forensic medicine is a practical science bridging the law and medicine, which are the eyes of the society. It is nothing but the conglomeration of all the branches and specialties of medical science, which can be, simply defined as medical aspects of law.

Forensic medicine deals with the application of medical knowledge to aid in the administration of justice through law courts.

(Forensic open forum → debating place—court of law)

Medical jurisprudence (Juris—law, prudentia—knowledge) deals with legal aspects of medical practice governing the duties and responsibilities of the medical practitioner to the patient and to the state.

Medical ethics deals with the code of principles that guide the members of the medical profession in dealings with their patients, their colleagues and also to the state safely.

Medical etiquette deals with the conventional laws of courtesy to be observed among the members of the medical profession.

Forensic medicine is broadly divided into

1. Clinical forensic medicine deals with medical examination of living individuals for legal purposes.
2. Forensic thanatology deals with medicolegal aspects of death in detail.
3. Forensic toxicology deals with clinical, analytical and circumstantial aspects of poisons.

Apart from this major division each and every branch of medical science is contributing to this speciality and in turn the entire medical profession is governed and guarded by this subject. The following are some of the important scientific subdivisions also contributing to forensic medicine.

- Forensic anthropology
- Forensic odontology
- Forensic serology
- Forensic ballistics
- Forensic psychiatry
- Forensic immunology, etc.

Practical is nothing but application of theoretical knowledge to solve problem whenever required with great skill and care.

Quotes

"Forensic medicine is a sanctuary for the victims of violence and treachery should have no part in the practice."

"Honesty dispensed with compassion is an integral part of truth and truth is nothing but justice in action to the people in need and distress."

"For murder though it has no tongue
Will speak with the most miraculous organ"

—*Shakespeare (Hamlet)*

"Truth is incontrovertible,
Panic may resent it.
Ignorance may deride it.
Malice may distort it
But there it is."

—*Winston Churchill*

"Dead body never tell lies unlike the living"
"Each dead body is a textbook which teaches the living "
"If the law has made you a witness remain a man of science since
You have no enemy to avenge or friend to save "

Clinical Forensic Medicine

Clinical forensic medicine deals with medicolegal examination of living persons. It should be done only under written authorization of an appropriate law enforcement authority. Written informed consent from the individual should be obtained and irrespective of the nature of the alleged offence and the type of examination to be done. Certain precautions and requirements are mandatory before commencing the examination.

Five most important information to be gathered and documented before examination for the purpose of positive identification of the individual at a later date and also to prevent false charges of criminal force leveled against the doctor (Sections 352 and 354 IPC).

1. Time, date and place of examination
2. Name, age, sex, address and occupation of the individual to be examined.
3. Victim/accused brought by whom, if police, rank or number with name and police station or if by relative, name and nature of relationship.
4. At least two identification marks preferably over the exposed parts of the body.
5. Written informed consent of the individual/guardian.

Consent

Definition

Consent can be defined as voluntary submission of an individual of sound mind and competent age to undergo certain examination.

The principle of consent was summed up by the great American Jurist Cardozo as follows.

"Every human being of adult years and sound mind has a right to determine what shall be done with his/her own body."

Consent in medical practice: In the context of medical practice, the following situations are concerned with consent.

Living Individuals

1. Medical examination: Diagnostic and therapeutic
2. Medicolegal examination: Legal purposes

Dead Bodies

1. Medicolegal/Pathological
2. Cadaver organ donation

Types of Consent

A. Implied consent
B. Expressed consent
   1. Verbal or Oral
   2. Written
C. Informed consent

Rules of Consent

IPC 87: 18 years is the age of consent for acts with inherent risk of death or hurt.

IPC 88: No offence when an act done under valid consent, not intended to cause death and for the persons benefit.

IPC 89: Consent of the guardian is necessary for a child under 12 years or for an insane person

IPC 90: Consent obtained by force or threat is not valid

IPC 91: Consent for an illegal act is not valid

IPC 92: Consent is not necessary in emergency life saving procedures.

IPC 93: Communications made in good faith and for the benefit of the person is not an offence.

Age Estimation

Ageing is a process that begins at conception and continues as long as we live. At any given time age can be estimated throughout our lifespan by various parameters and even after death it can be estimated from the remains.

Age is an important preliminary ingredient in all medicolegal examinations especially in personal identification.

- **What is age?**
  Age is the length of time that a person has existed since birth.
- **What is chronological age?**
  Chronological age is the length of time that elapsed since birth of an individual, expressed in measure of units usually in months or years.

  or

  Chronological age is the age of an individual measured in units of time usually in months/years since birth.
- **What is biological age?**
  Biological age refers to the age of a person estimated on the basis of growth and development in comparison with normal standards.
- **Need for age determination:**
  When birth is not registered (no Birth Certificate).
  Fake Birth Certificate (disputed Birth Certificate).
  Documents other than a Birth Certificate (School Leaving Certificate) is not available.
  When there is a gross difference between visual age and stated age.
- **Methods of age determination**
  Determination of age is based on the development and maturation of various biological systems during growth phase. The four maturity indicators useful in determining the biological age of an individual are:
  1. Somatic maturation — Progressive change in size and shape.
  2. Dental maturation — Dental development and eruption pattern.
  3. Sexual maturation — Development of secondary sexual characteristics
  4. Skeletal maturation — Development of complete bone from cartilaginous mould through ossification process at various site at specific periods of growth.

Somatic Maturation

Physical examination to estimate the age is more useful in foetus, infant, childhood and in adolescent period.

The important data for physical examination are
1. Height
2. Weight
3. Appearance and distribution of hair
4. Secondary sexual characteristics
5. Senile changes

Growth is an essential feature that starts from the time of conception until the child grows into a matured adult.

1. Height

Height at birth	50 cm
Height at 3 months	60 cm
Height at 9 months	70 cm
Height at 12 months	75 cm
Height at 24 months	90 cm
Height at 48 months	100 cm

From 4 to 10 years the height increases by 5 cm/year.

Stem stature index is the ratio between crown-rump length and crown-heel length. Infantometer is useful to measure the sitting height and standing height of an infant.

$$\text{Stem stature index} = \frac{\text{Crown-rump length}}{\text{Crown-heel length}} \times 100$$

At birth and up to 6 months	67%
1 year	64%
2 years	61%
3 years	58%
5 years	55%
10 years	52%

Head circumference:

At birth	35 cm
3 months	40 cm
1 year	45 cm
2 years	48 cm
7 years	50 cm
10 years	52 cm

2. Weight

At birth	2.5 to 3 kg
At 5 months	Two times the birth weight
At 1 year	Three times the birth weight
At 2 years	Four times the birth weight
At 5 years	Birth weight multiplied by 6
At 10 years	Birth weight multiplied by 10

Mean Height and Weight in Indian Girls

Age in years	Mean height in cm	Average ± 2 SD in cm	Mean weight in kg	Average ± 2 SD in kg
6	118	107–128	20	15–28
7	120	109–131	22	16–30
8	126	114–138	24	16–36
9	132	119–145	28	20–42
10	138	124–152	37	22–50
11	144	130–158	39	25–56
12	151	137–165	41	27–63
13	159	145–172	46	31–65
14	160	147–174	50	35–70
15	161	148–175	54	35–72
16	162	149–175	55	39–75
17	163	150–175	56	41–80
18	163–164	151–175	57	42–80

Mean Height and Weight in Indian Boys

Age in years	Mean height in cm	Average ± 2 SD in cm	Mean weight in kg	Average ± 2 SD in kg
6	116	106–125	21	16–26
7	121	112–132	23	18–30
8	127	116–138	26	19–35
9	132	120–143	28	21–40
10	138	125–150	31	22–46
11	146	132–161	35	23–49
12	150	135–160	40	27–60
13	157	140–173	45	30–67
14	163	146–180	51	35–75
15	169	152–185	57	40–82
16	174	160–188	62	45–88
17	176	163–189	66	49–95
18	177	164–190	69	51–97

Sexual Maturation

• Puberty:

10–14 years: Female

12–17 years: Male

• Pubertal changes:

Female:	Breast development [Thelarche]	8–12 years
	Pubic hair growth [Pubarche]	12–14 years
	Onset of menstruation [Menarche]	12–14 years
	Axillary hair growth	13–15 years
Male:	Enlargement of penis and testicles	12–14 years
	Pubic hair growth	13–15 years
	Axillary hair	14–16 years
	Facial hair	16–18 years
	Change in voice	14–17 years

Fast growth occurs after puberty until growth ceases at 25 years

• Post adult—Senile (degenerative) changes

Greying of hair, Balding	after 40 years
Skin wrinkles over the face	after 50 years
Arcus senilis cataract	after 60 years
Osteoporotic changes	after 60 years
Skull suture obliteration	after 70 years

Dictum in Age Estimation

Childhood	By physical and dental examination
Adolescence	By sexual development, dental and radiological examination
Adult	Skull (sutural fusion), sternum—fusion (body with manubrium and xiphi sternum)
Old age	Degenerative changes/osteoporosis

The age can be estimated almost accurately when the person is young (range—two years) and the range of age gets wider as the person grows older (range—five to ten years).

Physical maturation should always be corroborated with dental maturation and/or skeletal maturation to determine the age near accuracy in reasonable range.

Hippocratic Oath

The Hippocratic Oath is an oath historically taken by doctors swearing to practice medicine ethically. It is widely believed to have been written by Hippocrates, the Father of Western Medicine. A widely used modern version of the traditional oath was penned in 1964 by Dr. Louis Lasagna, former Principal of Sackler School of Graduate Biomedical Sciences and Academic Dean of the School of Medicine at Tufts University.

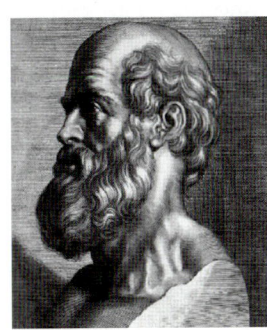

Original

Original, translated into English:

I swear by *Apollo*, the healer, *Asclepius, Hygieia*, and *Panacea*, and I take to witness all the gods, all the goddesses, to keep according to my ability and my judgment, the following oath and agreement:

To consider dear to me, as my parents, him who taught me *this art*; to live in common with him and, if necessary, to share my goods with him; to look upon his children as my own brothers, to teach them this art.

I will *prescribe* regimens for the good of my patients according to my ability and my judgment and *never do harm* to anyone.

I will not *give a lethal drug to anyone if I am asked*, nor will I advise such a plan; and similarly I will not give a woman a *pessary* to cause an *abortion*.

But I will preserve the purity of my life and my arts.

I will not *cut for stone*, even for patients in whom the disease is manifest; I will leave this operation to be performed by practitioners, specialists in *this art*.

In every house where I come I will enter only for the good of my patients, keeping myself far from all intentional ill-doing and all seduction and especially from the pleasures of love with women or with men, be they free or slaves.

All that may come to my knowledge in the exercise of my profession or in daily commerce with men, which ought not to be spread abroad, I will *keep secret* and will never reveal.

If I keep this oath faithfully, may I enjoy my life and practice my art, respected by all men and in all times; but if I *swerve* from it or violate it, may the reverse be my lot.

Modern Version

I swear to fulfill, to the best of my ability and judgment, this covenant: I will respect the hard-won scientific gains of those physicians in whose steps I walk, and gladly share such knowledge as is mine with those who are to follow.

I will apply, for the benefit of the sick, all measures [that] are required, avoiding those twin traps of overtreatment and therapeutic nihilism.

I will remember that there is art to medicine as well as science, and that warmth, sympathy, and understanding may outweigh the surgeon's knife or the chemist's drug.

I will not be ashamed to say "I know not," nor will I fail to call in my colleagues when the skills of another are needed for a patient's recovery.

I will respect the privacy of my patients, for their problems are not disclosed to me that the world may know. Most especially must I tread with care in matters of life and death. If it is given to me to save a life, all thanks. But it may also be within my power to take a life; this awesome responsibility must be faced with great humbleness and awareness of my own frailty. Above all, I must not play at God.

I will remember that I do not treat a fever chart, a cancerous growth, but a sick human being, whose illness may affect the person's family and economic stability. My responsibility includes these related problems, if I am to care adequately for the sick.

I will prevent disease whenever I can, for prevention is preferable to cure.

I will remember that I remain a member of society, with special obligations to all my fellow human beings, those sound of mind and body as well as the infirm.

If I do not violate this oath, may I enjoy life and art, respected while I live and remembered with affection thereafter. May I always act so as to preserve the finest traditions of my calling and may I long experience the joy of healing those who seek my help.

Clinical
Forensic Medicine

Section
1

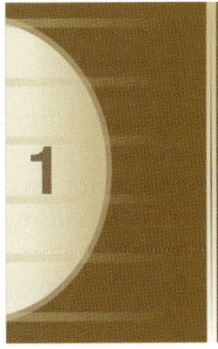

1

Age Estimation by Dental Examination

INTRODUCTION

As the knowledge of development, eruption and morphological anatomy of teeth is essential for a better application in forensic practice, dental examination has been described briefly in this chapter.

All the teeth do not develop at the same rate, hence the eruption also occurs at different times. Likewise not all the primary or deciduous teeth are lost simultaneously. The twenty primary teeth erupt into the oral cavity in a span of 2 or 2½ years from 6th month onwards after birth. This primary tooth remains only for a short period because they are replaced with their corresponding succedaneous or permanent teeth in a regular sequence as the child grows.

The first temporary or primary tooth, the central incisor erupts first followed by lateral incisor, first primary molar, primary canine and second primary molar lastly. Like their sequential eruption, the exfoliation also occurs in the same order of sequence in a span of 6 years from 6th year onwards.

At the age of 6th year the first permanent molar appears in the oral cavity. At the same time the primary central incisor falls off. The second permanent molar erupts usually at 12th year. In the period between 6th and 12th years all the primary teeth are replaced with their corresponding permanent teeth in a fairly regular sequence. During the interval between the eruption of first and second permanent molars (6 years to 12 years), both temporary and permanent teeth can be seen in the oral cavity of an individual. Hence this period (6–12 years) is known as *mixed dentition period* or *transitional period*. During this transitional period all the primary teeth are replaced by permanent teeth followed by the eruption of second permanent molar between 12 and 14 years and finally the third molar between 17 and 25 years.

Dental maturation is accepted as one of the best maturity indicators which involves two separate processes. One is dental development (mineralisation) and the other is dental emergence (eruption). The former can be assessed with the help of suitable radiographs and the later can be done by counting the number of erupted teeth in the oral cavity.

TOOTH DEVELOPMENT

A tooth undergoes different maturation stages. Initially it starts with the formation of crypt and ends with apical closure. During this maturation process there is a progressive change in size and shape of the tooth. The developmental period for the temporary teeth extends from

3rd month of intrauterine life to third year of postnatal life and for the permanent teeth the developmental period extends from 6th month to 16 years of age.

The alveolar sockets which hold the teeth are formed around the third or fourth month of intrauterine life. Development of tooth begins with the formation of cellular tooth germs within the alveolar bone, in the shape of the crown. Apposition and calcification of enamel and dentine occur within this germ tooth. The crown is completely formed and calcified before any positional changes occur. At birth, the rudiments of all the temporary and their corresponding permanent (40) teeth along with the first permanent molars (4) are found in both the jaws. Root formation begins after completion of the crown. As the root becomes longer the crown erupts through the bone and the overlying gum and finally emerges into the oral cavity. The root is completed after the tooth is fully functional. During eruption of the permanent tooth, the overlying root of its deciduous predecessor undergoes resorption, until the crown only remains and the unsupported crown finally falls. In that gap the permanent counterpart erupts. The eruption of teeth is variable depending on heredity, environment, nutrition and endocrine function, but the development of teeth is less affected by these factors.

A tooth is a combination of compliment from ectoderm, mesoderm and endoderm. The enamel is derived from ectoderm of the oral cavity; all other tissues from the surrounding mesenchyme and neural crest cells. The development is divided into different stages for descriptive purpose based on the appearance of the developing tooth—buds that appear in the anterior mandibular region first, next in the anterior maxillary region and then progress posteriorly to both jaws.

Bud Stage of Tooth Development

Tooth development begins in the 6th week of intrauterine life as a thickening of oral ectoderm over the curves of the primordial mandibular and maxillary arches. This thickened oral epithelium is known as dental lamina (Fig. 1.1). Each dental lamina develops 10 centers of proliferation of ectoderm from which swellings—**tooth buds** (tooth germs) (Fig. 1.2)—grow into the underlying mesenchyme. These buds develop into **deciduous teeth**. The tooth buds for **permanent teeth** that have deciduous predecessors begin to appear from deep continuation of the dental lamina. They develop lingual to the **deciduous tooth buds**. The permanent molars have no deciduous predecessors and develop as buds from posterior extensions of the **dental laminae**. The buds for the second and third permanent molars develop only after birth.

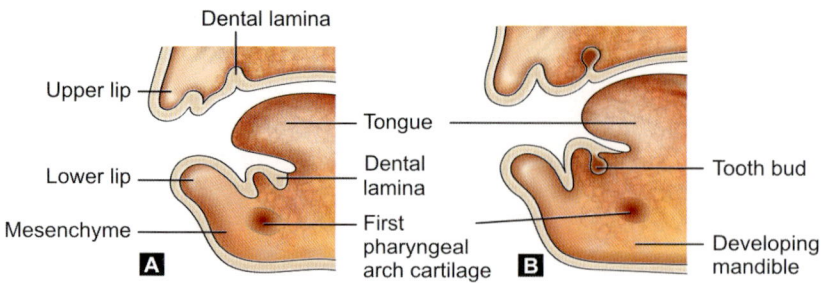

Fig. 1.1: Ectodermal thickening and growth

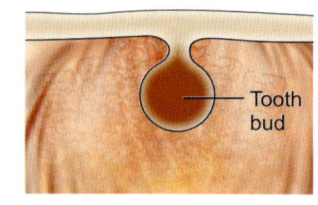

Fig. 1.2: Tooth bud invagination

Cap Stage of Tooth Development

The ectodermal part of the developing tooth, the **enamel organ** (Fig. 1.3) eventually produces enamel. The internal part of each cap-shaped tooth is the **dental papilla.** Together, the dental papilla and enamel organ form the tooth bud. The *outer cell layer* of the enamel organ is the **outer enamel epithelium**, and the *inner cell layer* lining the papilla is the **inner enamel epithelium**. The core between the layers of enamel epithelium is the **enamel reticulum** (stellate reticulum). As the enamel organ and dental papilla of the tooth develop, the mesenchyme surrounding the developing tooth condenses to form the **dental sac.** The dental sac is the primordium of the *cement and periodontal ligament.* The **cement** is the bonelike connective tissue covering the root of the tooth. The **periodontal ligament** is the fibrous connective tissue that surrounds the root of the tooth, which anchors the tooth strongly to the alveolar bone.

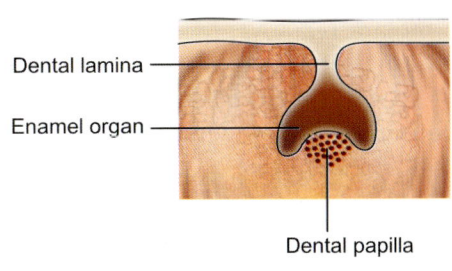

Dental lamina

Enamel organ

Dental papilla

Fig. 1.3: Cap stage

Bell Stage of Tooth Development

The mesenchymal cells in the dental papilla adjacent to the internal enamel epithelium (Fig. 1.4) differentiate into **odontoblasts**, which produce predentine. Later, the **predentine** calcifies and becomes dentine, the second hardest tissue in the body. As the dentine thickens, the odontoblasts regress toward the center of the dental papilla. Enamel is the hardest tissue in the body. It overlies and protects the dentine from being fractured.

Cells of the *inner enamel epithelium* (Fig. 1.4) differentiate into ameloblasts under the influence of the odontoblast, which produces enamel in the form of prisms over the dentine. As the enamel increases, the ameloblasts migrate toward the *outer enamel epithelium*. Enamel and dentine formation begin at the cusp of the tooth and progress toward the future root.

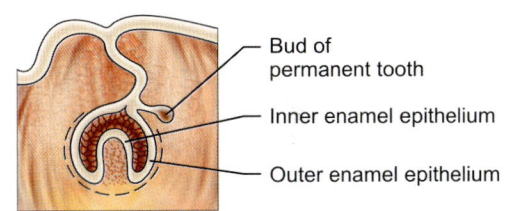

Bud of permanent tooth

Inner enamel epithelium

Outer enamel epithelium

Fig. 1.4: Bell stage

The **root of the tooth** begins to develop after dentine and enamel formation are well advanced. The inner and outer enamel epithelia fuse together in the **neck of the tooth** (cement-enamel junction), where they form a fold, the **epithelial root sheath**. This sheath grows into the mesenchyme and initiates root formation. The *odontoblasts* adjacent to the epithelial root sheath form dentine that is continuous with that of the crown. As the dentine increases, it reduces the **pulp cavity** to a narrow **root canal** through which the vessels and nerves pass. The inner cells of the dental sac differentiate into **cementoblasts**, which produce cement that is restricted to the root. Cement is deposited over the dentine of the root and meets the enamel at the neck of the tooth.

As the teeth develop each tooth soon becomes surrounded by bone, except over its crown. The tooth is held in its **alveolus** by the strong **periodontal ligament**, a derivative of the dental sac. The periodontal ligament is located between the cement of the root and the bony alveolus.

TOOTH MORPHOLOGY

Man is gifted with two sets of teeth. The first set erupts in the oral cavity during childhood and the second set erupts during late childhood and adolescent period. The first set exists for a short period, hence it is termed *temporary or primary or deciduous teeth* and the second set remains permanent unless worn out, hence it is termed *permanent or succedaneous teeth*.

The total numbers of temporary teeth are 20 (5 in each quadrant—2 incisors, 1 canine, 2 molars I–2, C–1, M–2). The total numbers of permanent teeth are 32 (8 in each quadrant — 2 incisors, 1 canine, 2 premolars, 3 molars, I–2, C–1, PM–2, M–3).

Irrespective of the type, each tooth erupts at a particular age and this forms the basis of age determination by dental eruption.

As per the development and eruption, the permanent teeth are divided into two types.

1. **Successional permanent teeth** are those which erupt in place occupied by deciduous teeth. Successional teeth are ten in each jaw.
2. **Superadded permanent teeth** are those which do not have corresponding deciduous predecessors. They erupt behind the temporary teeth. All the permanent molars are superadded permanent teeth (six in each jaw).

Incisors

The anterior biting teeth are 8 in numbers, the crown is shovel shaped and has an incisal edge and the root is conical and single. The maxillary incisors are larger than mandibular incisors. The sharp, chisel-shaped front teeth (four upper and four lower) are used for cutting food (Fig. 1.5).

Canine

They are stronger and longer than any other teeth and have a pointed cusp and a long single root. In total 4 canines are present, one in each quadrant. Sometimes called cuspids, these teeth are shaped like points (or cusps) and are used for tearing food (Fig. 1.5).

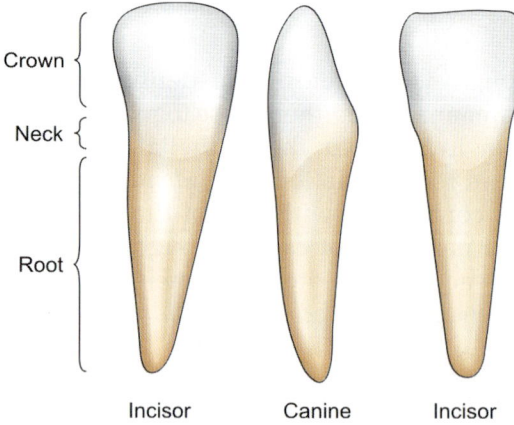

Crown

Neck

Root

Incisor   Canine   Incisor

Fig. 1.5: Cuspids

Premolars

They are present only in permanent teeth which erupt in the place of temporary molars. They are 8 in number, 2 in each quadrant. Crown is oval shaped having two cusps (bicuspid). All premolars are single rooted except the maxillary first premolar which has two roots (Fig. 1.6). These teeth have two pointed cusps on their biting surface and are sometimes referred to as bicuspids. The premolars are used for crushing and tearing of food.

Molars

The number of deciduous molar is 8 (2 in each quadrant), whereas the number of permanent molars is 12 (3 in each quadrant). Crowns of all the molars have more than 3 or 4 cusps (Fig. 1.7). Root of maxillary molars is three in number, whereas the root of mandibular molars is two. The first mandibular molars are the largest among all teeth. Molars are used for grinding the food.

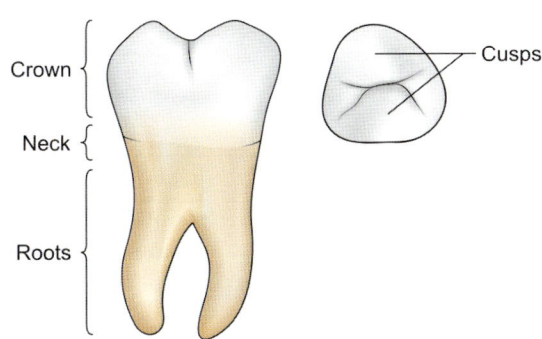

Fig. 1.6: Premolar (bicuspid)

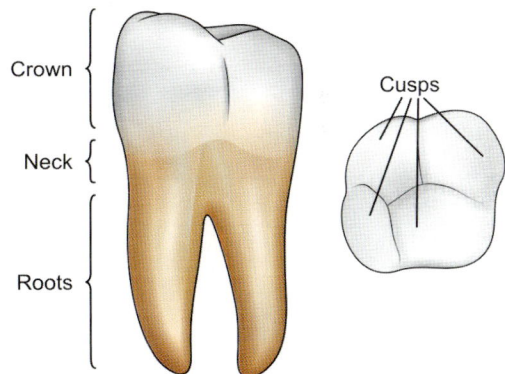

Fig. 1.7: Molar (four cusps)

TEMPORARY TEETH ERUPTION (TABLE 1.1)

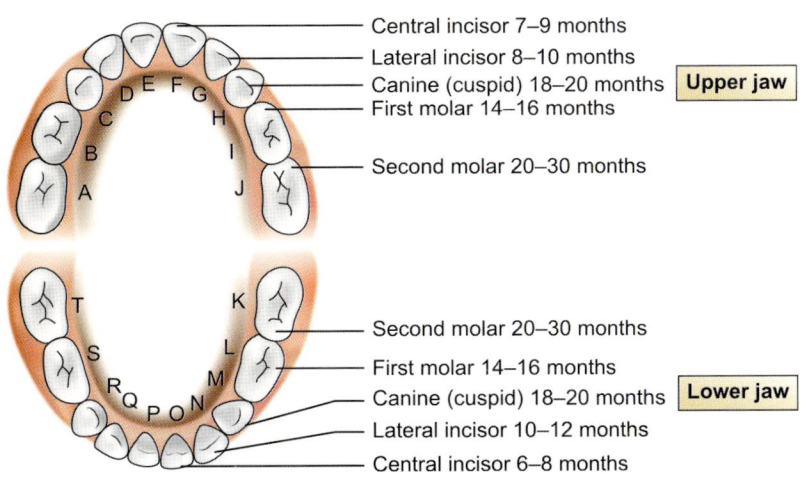

Central incisor 7–9 months
Lateral incisor 8–10 months
Canine (cuspid) 18–20 months **Upper jaw**
First molar 14–16 months

Second molar 20–30 months

Second molar 20–30 months
First molar 14–16 months
Canine (cuspid) 18–20 months **Lower jaw**
Lateral incisor 10–12 months
Central incisor 6–8 months

Fig. 1.8: Temporary tooth eruption

PERMANENT TEETH ERUPTION (TABLE 1.2)

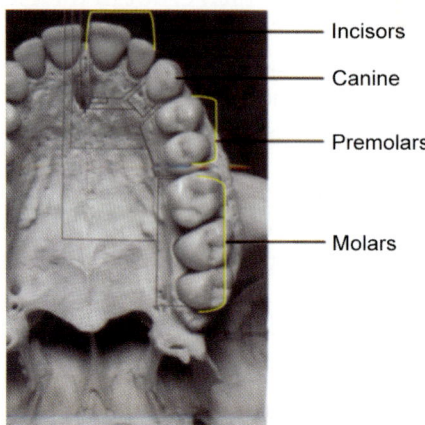

Incisors

Canine

Premolars

Molars

Fig. 1.9: Permanent teeth (maxilla)

Table 1.1: Eruption of temporary tooth

Tooth	Age of eruption
Central incisor	
Lower	6 to 8 months
Upper	7 to 9 months
Lateral incisor	
Upper	8 to 10 months
Lower	10 to 12 months
First molar	12 to 14 months
Canine	16 to 18 months
Second molar	20 to 30 months

Table 1.2: Eruption of permanent tooth

Tooth	Eruption time
Central incisor	6–8 years
Lateral incisor	7–9 years
Canine	11–12 years
First premolar	9–11 years
Second premolar	10–12 years
First molar	6–7 years
Second molar	12–14 years
Third molar	17–25 years

DIFFERENCE BETWEEN TEMPORARY AND PERMANENT TEETH

In children between 6 and 12 years both deciduous and permanent teeth can be seen in the oral cavity (Figs 1.10 and 1.11) and the developing permanent counterparts are seen behind each primary

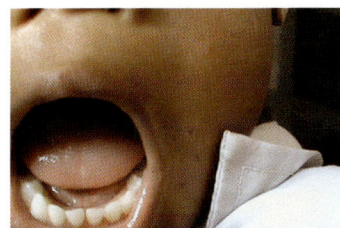

Fig. 1.10: Temporary teeth

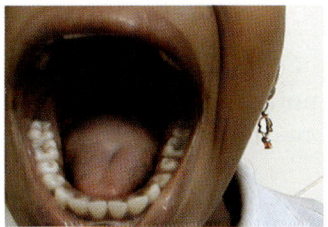

Fig. 1.11: Permanent teeth

tooth in an orthopantomography (OPG). Hence knowledge of differences between deciduous and permanent teeth is essential for determining age accurately or near to accuracy (Table 1.3).

Table 1.3: Differences between temporary and permanent teeth

Character	Temporary	Permanent
1. Numbers	20	32
2. Eruption period	From 6 months to 30 months	6 years to 25 years
3. Size	Small	Large
4. Shape	Bulbous with prominent neck	Not so
5. Colour	Milky white	Dull white
6. Direction	Vertical	Inclined (anteriorly)
7. Type	Premolars absent	8 premolars present
8. Formula	$I_2C_1M_2$	$I_2C_1P_2M_3$ (in each quadrant)
9. Root (molar)	More divergent	Normal
10. Life span	Limited (only up to 12 years)	Unlimited (worn out due to ageing)

Teeth Eruption

As the **deciduous teeth** develop, they begin a continuous slow movement towards the oral cavity. This process called **eruption** results in emergence of the tooth from its developmental position in the jaw to its functional position in the mouth. The **mandibular teeth** usually erupt before the **maxillary teeth** and teeth in girls usually erupt earlier than boys. Usually eruption of the deciduous teeth occur between the 6th and 24th months after birth roughly 6 months apart between each type of teeth (i.e. incisors—6 months, first molar—12 months, canine—18 months, second molar—24 months). All 20 deciduous teeth are usually present by the end of second year in healthy children. The complete permanent dentition consists of 32 teeth. As a permanent tooth grows, the root of the overlying deciduous tooth is gradually resorbed by **osteoclasts** (odontoclasts). Consequently, it consists only of the crown which is later shed. The permanent teeth usually begin to erupt during the sixth year and continue to appear until early adulthood. The permanent teeth that erupt in the space occupied by deciduous (anterior 20) teeth are called successional permanent teeth and the permanent teeth that erupt in the space not occupied by deciduous (posterior 12) teeth called superadded permanent (all molars) teeth.

From examination of OPG picture, the eruption takes places in three phases—alveolar, gingival and functional.

DENTAL NOTATIONS—GUSTAFSON'S FORMULA

To document the dentition of an individual, several notations are used.

1. **Szigmondy notation**: The permanent teeth are given Arabic numerals and temporary teeth are given Roman numerals from mesial to distal side in all quadrants of both the jaws as follows.

Permanent

Szigmondy notation

R   L

R															L
8	7	6	5	4	3	2	1	1	2	3	4	5	6	7	8
8	7	6	5	4	3	2	1	1	2	3	4	5	6	7	8

Temporary

V	IV	III	II	I	I	II	III	IV	V
V	IV	III	II	I	I	II	III	IV	V

2. **Cunningham notation (universal system):** In this notation the permanent teeth are indicated by Arabic numerals from 1 to 32, whereas the Roman numerals are replaced with 20 english letters from A to T in clockwise manner from right upper to right lower quadrant across left upper and left lower quadrant.

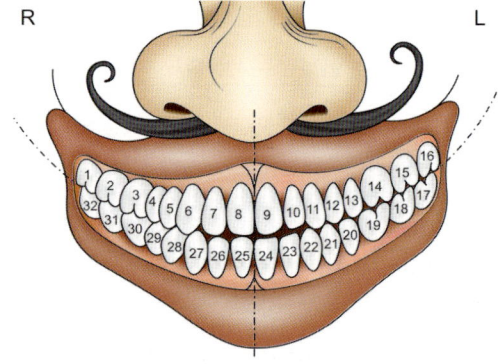

Cunningham notation

Permanent

RU															LU
1	2	3	4	5	6	7	8	9	10	11	12	13	14	15	16
32	31	30	29	28	27	26	25	24	23	22	21	20	19	18	17
RL															LL

Temporary

A	B	C	D	E	F	G	H	I	J
T	S	R	Q	P	O	N	M	L	K

3. **Navy notation:** The digits and letters start from right side of each jaw.

Permanent

								Navy notation							
RU															LU
1	2	3	4	5	6	7	8	9	10	11	12	13	14	15	16
17	18	19	20	21	22	23	24	25	26	27	28	29	30	31	32
RL															LL

Temporary

A	B	C	D	E	F	G	H	I	J
K	L	M	N	O	P	Q	R	S	T

4. **Palmer notation:** The permanent teeth are given with Arabic numerals as in Szigmondy notation but the temporary teeth are awarded english letters from A to E.

Permanent

							Palmer notation							
R														L
8	7	6	5	4	3	2	1	1	2	3	4	5	6	7	8
8	7	6	5	4	3	2	1	1	2	3	4	5	6	7	8

Temporary

E	D	C	B	A	A	B	C	D	E
E	D	C	B	A	A	B	C	D	E

5. **Federation of dentaire international (FDI):** As per this FDI notation each tooth is awarded with a double digit number, the right digit indicates the quadrant of the mouth cavity and generic type of tooth and the left digit indicates the position of the tooth in the jaw from midline to posterior. The advantages of this FDI formula over the others are (a) the necessity to specify the quadrant does not arise, (b) both temporary and permanent teeth can be recorded in the same notation.

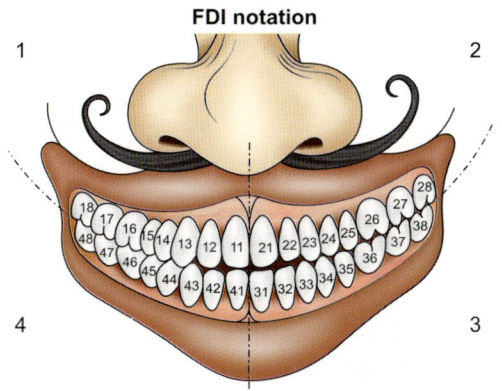

FDI notation

First fix the number according to the position occupied by each tooth from mesial to distal in all four quadrants. Now add the second digit in front of the existing numbers, 1 to 4 in case of permanent and 5 to 8 in case of temporary in clockwise manner from right upper to right lower quadrant across the left upper and left lower quadrants.

Permanent

RU   LU

18	17	16	15	14	13	12	11	21	22	23	24	25	26	27	28
48	47	46	45	44	43	42	41	31	32	33	34	35	36	37	38

RL   LL

Temporary

55	54	53	52	51	61	62	63	64	65
85	84	83	82	81	71	72	73	74	75

Gustafson's Formula

Age estimation by Gustafson's formula is based on the following wear and tear changes that affect the teeth of adults.

1. Attrition   0 : No change
2. Paradentosis   1 : Mild change
3. Secondary dentine   2 : Moderate change
4. Root resorption   3 : Severe change
5. Transparency of root
6. Cementum apposition
   (point value)   A3 + P3 + S3+ R3 + T3 + C3 = 18

Each factor is described in 4 degrees starting from 0 to 4. By summing up all the changes, the point value is calculated and with this point value the age can be determined using regression charts. Of all the changes root transparency is most reliable.

Procedure of Examination

Examination of age can be carried out only after implied consent of the individual. The procedure is conveniently done in 3 stages

1. Examination
2. Documentation and
3. Certification

Step 1: Examine the dental pattern with a torch with widely opened mouth without causing discomfort to the individual.

or

Read the given problem (if there is no volunteer to examine) more than once or examine the maxillary part of the cranium or the given mandible or dental cast.

Step 2: Count the total number of **erupted** teeth in the oral cavity as well as the space where the tooth/teeth has fallen off.

or

If *X*-ray oblique view of mandible or OPG is given, examine it (in case no volunteer is there to examine).

Step 3: Apply total number formula for approximate age estimation.

    (a) If the total number of erupted teeth is 20, it indicates all of them are primary or temporary or deciduous teeth and the age is less than 6 years (primary dentition period).

    (b) If the total number of erupted teeth is more than 20 but less than 24, it indicates presence of both temporary and permanent dentition, then the age is greater than 6 years and less than 12 years (mixed dentition period or transitional period).

    (c) If the teeth are more than 24 but less than 28, then the age is above 12 years.

    (d) If the total number of teeth is more than 28, then the age is above 17 years.

Step 4: After assessing the approximate age by total number formula, now apply individual tooth eruption formula for assessment of age with reasonable or acceptable range of two years as follows:

Figure 1.12 shows the OPG of a child. Total number of teeth in the oral cavity is 20, i.e. 5 in each quadrant. The first permanent molar is not erupted and the second molar is developing and developing permanent teeth are seen behind the temporary teeth. This shows the age to be less than 6 years.

Particular attention should be given during the mixed dentition period as both primary and permanent teeth are present, and the approximate age has to be assessed by total number of temporary and permanent teeth as given in Table 1.4.

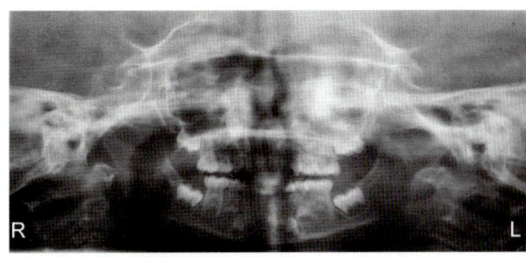

Fig. 1.12: OPG of a child less than 6 years

Apart from this total number of teeth, the difference between primary molars and premolars is very important. The most important morphological difference lies in the cusps and root. The molars are provided with more than three cusps and are bigger than the premolars which are provided with only two cusps (bicuspid) and are smaller in size. The root can be visualized in an X-ray as two for molars and one for premolars.

Table 1.4: Total number formula			
Total no. of teeth	*Temporary*	*Permanent*	*Approximate age in years*
24	20	4	Above 6 years
24	12	12	9 years
24	4	20	11 years
24	0	24	Above 12 years

The eruption of first permanent molar initiate the exfoliation of temporary teeth and the eruption of second permanent molar complete the exfoliation with loss of primary canines lastly.

In Figure 1.13, OPG showing 24 erupted tooth in the oral cavity. Of the 24, 12 are temporary (canine, first and second molar) and 12 are permanent (central and lateral incisors and permanent first molar). Age is above 7 years and below 9 years.

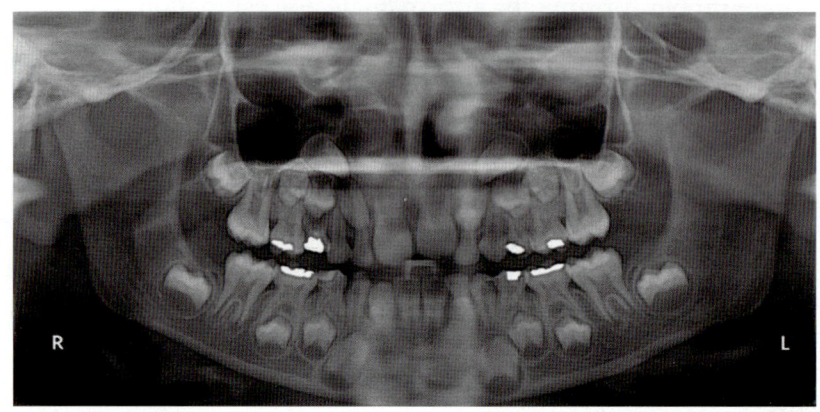

Fig. 1.13: OPG of a child of 7–9 years

For the final assessment, the lower limit of the range must be fixed with the latest erupted tooth and the upper limit of the range must be fixed with the unerupted tooth next in eruption sequence.

One must always remember that there is a long interval between the eruption of second permanent molar (12–14 years) and third permanent molar (17–25 years), so the range of dental age is wider which is neither appreciable nor applicable. To avoid this inconvenience, a physical examination involving the appearance of secondary sexual characteristics, i.e. hair growth over the pubis, axilla and face (in male) is more useful than the development of genitals and breast (female) to corroborate with the dental age within a reasonable and acceptable range.

Pubic hair commenced at 12 years and completed (adult) at 14 years

Axillary hair commenced at 14 years and completed at 16 years

Facial hair commenced at 16 years and completed at 18 years (male)

Space for third molar by elongation of jaw seen after 16 years

In Fig. 1.14, the OPG shows all permanent teeth with functional eruption of second molar also. The third molar in all the quadrants show only alveolar eruption. Hence the lower limit of range of age is twelve years and the upper limit can be fixed with appearance of hair growth over the pubic region as 14 years as shown in Fig. 1.15, since the pubic hair has just commenced to appear.

In Fig. 1.16, the OPG shows all permanent teeth with functional eruption of second molar also. The third molar in all the quadrants show only alveolar eruption. However, the pubic hair is fully grown (Fig. 1.17) and axillary hair growth has started in this individual. Hence the age is above 14 years and below 16 years.

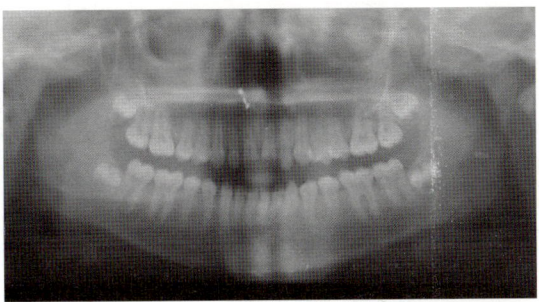

Fig. 1.14: OPG of a female above 12 years

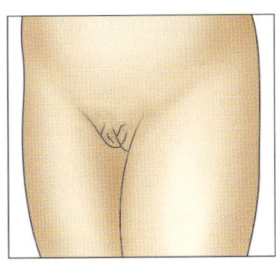

Fig. 1.15: Few black pubic hair in a child of 12–14 years

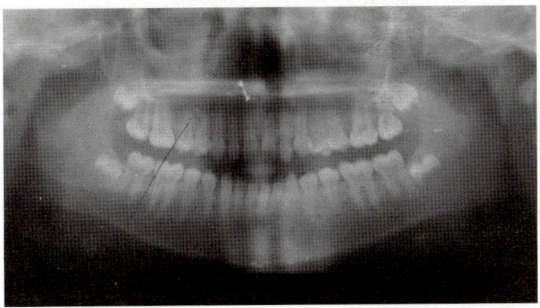

Fig. 1.16: OPG of a female of above 14 years

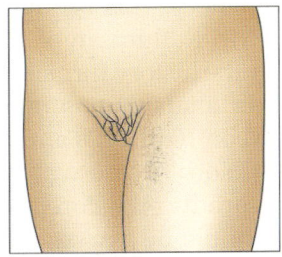

Fig. 1.17: Fully grown pubic hair above 14 years

Documentation

Documentation should be done step by step.

1. Serial number of age case.
2. Identity of the authorising officer with crime number, police station/court with date.
3. Identity of the escort police who brought the person with requisition.
4. Identity of the individual to be examined. Personal data name, age, sex, address and occupation.
5. Two identification marks
6. Consent
7. Time and date of examination
8. Physical findings:

   Height

   Weight

   Breadth

   Chest circumference — Full inspiration / Full expiration

   Abdominal girth (umbilical level)

9. Hair growth: Scalp, pubis, axilla, mustache, beard

10. Dental examination

           FDI Formula

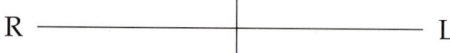

   R ————————————————— L

11. Opinion as to the age

     Date   Signature of the MO

     Place   with date

EXERCISE

On 11.01.2009, a boy named Suresh, S/O Shanmugam, a resident of No. 3, Kamaraj Nagar, Guduvanchery, was brought to the Department of Forensic Medicine, by Head Constable No.130, Mr. Kathiresan of Meenambakkam Police Station.

As per the history furnished by the Inspector of Police, Meenambakkam, Suresh was roaming around in a suspicious manner at the arrival hall of the Anna International Terminal at 01.30 AM on 10.01.2009 and he was secured by CISF personnel and handed over to the Airport Police Station. A case was registered on 10.01.2009 against him under Section 448 IPC. The boy was produced before the Judicial Magistrate, Chingleput and the Magistrate ordered that his age should be assessed; hence he was brought to the Department of Forensic Medicine.

The examination was conducted at 11 AM in the Department of Forensic Medicine on 11.01.2009 and following were the findings.

Moderately nourished adolescent with slightly broken voice.

Physical Findings

Height   —   135 cm
Weight   —   26 kg
Breadth   —   28 cm

Chest   ⟨ Normal—36 cm

         Full inspiration—40 cm

Abdominal girth   —   38 cm
Hair growth   —   Scalp black, 5 cm, facial hair not appeared
Pubis   —   A few downy hairs around root of penis.
Axilla   —   No hair

Dental Examination

Dental pattern given in OPG picture.

Identification Marks

1. A black mole on front of right side of the chest.
2. A black mole over the right side of neck.

    How will you proceed with the examination and give your opinion based on the dental data?

Register No.....................

Department of Forensic Medicine
Age Estimation Proforma

Requisition from The Judicial Magistrate of/Inspector of ....

vide letter/crime no. .... dated ....

1. Name of the individual   :
2. Sex   :
3. Parent's or guardian's name   :
4. Residential address   :
5. Occupation   :
6. Marital status   :
7. Age as alleged by
   (a) Individual to be examined   :
   (b) People or Police accompanying   :
8. Persons accompanying or brought by   :
9. Time, date and place of examination   :
10. Consent of the individual for examination   :
11. Signature of the individual consenting or his guardian   :
12. Marks of identification
    1.
    2.

Physical Examination

1. Height   :
2. Weight   :
3. Breadth   :
4. Chest girth at the level of the nipples   :
5. Abdominal girth at the level of the navel   :
6. General build and appearance   :
7. Voice   : Infantile/Broken/Adult
8. Teeth   : R ———————|——————— L
9. Hair   :
   Scalp
   Beard
   Moustache
   Axillary
   Pubic
10. Mammae—development   :
11. Generative organs—development   :
12. Date of menarche and regularity of cycle   :
13. Ossification   :
14. Opinion of age   :

Place   Professor of Forensic Medicine

Date:

Register No. ....

Department of Forensic Medicine
Age Certificate

From the Physical and Dental examination/Radiological examination of ....
.................S/o /D/o... resident of ....
.... bearing the
identification marks.

1.

2.

I am of the opinion that the individual is aged above .... years and below .... years.

Place

Date:

Signature

EVALUATORY QUESTIONS

1. **How important is assessment of age, in identification?**

   Age plays a vital role in establishing the identity of an individual. It is the most important preliminary requirement to trace a missing person or to identify a dead body.

2. **What is chronological age?**

   It is the length of time that has elapsed since the birth of an individual and is expressed in years and months.

   or

   Chronological Age is the age of an individual measured in units of time usually in years and months since birth.

3. **What is biological age?**

   Biological age refers to the age of a person estimated on the basis of growth and development in comparison with normal standards.

4. **What are the different indicators that are useful in age assessment?**

   The four important maturity indicators useful to assess the age of an individual are

   i.   Somatic maturation — Progressive change in size and shape.
   ii. Dental maturation — Dental development and eruption pattern.
   iii. Sexual maturation — Development of secondary sexual characteristics
   iv. Skeletal maturation — Development of complete bone from cartilaginous mould through ossification process at various sites at specific periods of growth.

5. **What is dental age?**

   It is the age of an individual estimated by development and eruption of teeth.

6. **What do you mean by mixed dentition?**

   Mixed dentition denotes the presence of both temporary and permanent teeth in the oral cavity of person.

7. **What is the normal period of mixed dentition?**
   The period of mixed dentition extends from the eruption of the first permanent molar to exfoliation of temporary canine tooth, i.e. from 6 years to 12 years.
8. **Which permanent tooth erupts first?**
   First molar
9. **Which temporary tooth falls off last?**
   The canine
10. **What is Gustafson's method?**
    Gustafson's method is useful in estimating the dental age of an adult with wear and tear dental changes.
11. **Which of the Gustafson factor is most dependable in age assessment?**
    Root transparency.

2 Age Estimation by Ossification

INTRODUCTION

The process of bone formation is known as ossification. The bones of the human and mammalian skeleton develop from a number of separate centres of ossification. Endochondral ossification starts in a small area at the middle of the shaft of the cartilagenous model during intrauterine life. This area is called the primary centre of ossification. At varying times after birth, the secondary centres of endochondral ossification appear in the cartilages forming the ends of the long bones, hence they are called secondary centres of ossification. After completion of ossification the ends of all the long bones (epiphyses) fuse with the shaft (diaphyses) at varying periods of growth.

It is estimated that at the eleventh prenatal week (11th week) in humans there are 806 centres of bone growth, at birth 450 centres, while the adult skeleton has only 206 bones. From the 11th prenatal week to the time of final union some 600 centres of bone growth "disappear"; that means they unite with adjacent centres to give rise to definite adult bones.

The process of appearance of ossification centres and union with the shaft occurs at a fairly definite sequence and time, and this makes it a reliable age indicator.

To appreciate the appearance and fusion of secondary ossification centres, ends of all long bones should be X-rayed. The joints of the upper and lower limbs comprise

1. *X*-ray shoulder
2. *X*-ray elbow
3. *X*-ray wrist
4. *X*-ray pelvis
5. *X*-ray knee
6. *X*-ray ankle

Apart from these normal sites, individuals who are nearing the cessation of growth, i.e. after 18 years, *X*-ray chest should be taken to view the medial end of clavicle and after 25 years *X*-ray of sternum in oblique view and *X*-ray skull in different views are taken for sutural fusion. Spinal column is *X*-rayed for appreciation of wear and tear of vertebral bodies.

ODD AND EVEN NUMBER FORMULAE OF EPIPHYSEAL FUSION

Even numbers [2, 4, 6]: Fusion between 14 and 16 years
Odd numbers [1, 3, 5]: Fusion between 16 and 18 years (Fig 2.1).

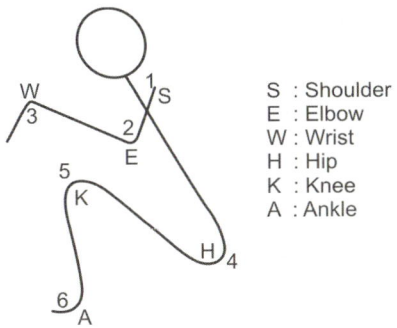

S : Shoulder
E : Elbow
W : Wrist
H : Hip
K : Knee
A : Ankle

Fig. 2.1: Odd and even number formulae

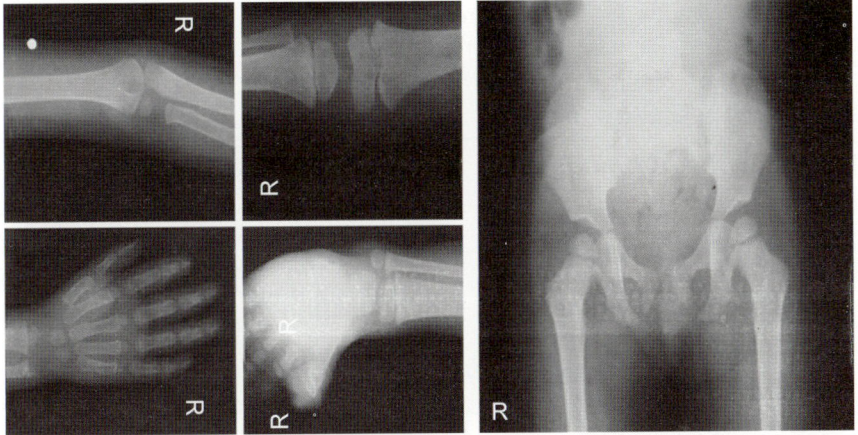

Fig. 2.2: X-rays of a child between 2 and 4 years

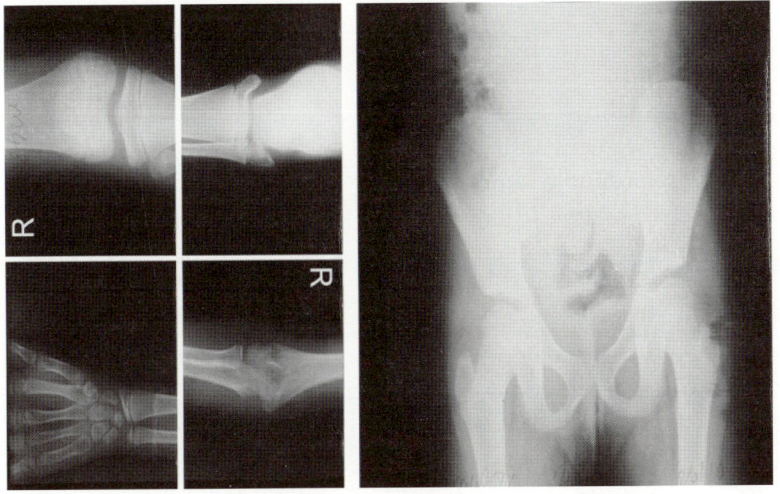

Fig. 2.3: X-rays of a child between 6 and 9 years

Appearance and Fusions of Ossification Centre

Table 2.1: Appearance and fusions of ossification centre

Name of joint	Ossification centre	Age of appearance	Age of fusion
1. X-ray shoulder AP view	1. Upper end of humerus		
	(a) Head	1st year ⎫ after 5 years	
	(b) Greater tubercle	2nd year ⎬ all fuses	16–18 years
	(c) Lesser tubercle	5th year ⎭ together	
	2. Acromion	14–16 years	18 years
	3. Coracoid process	3 years	16–18 years
2. X-ray Elbow AP view Lateral view	Capitulum ⎫	1 year	14–16 years
	Medial epicondyle ⎬ lower	5–7 years	16 years
	Trochlea ⎬ end of	9 years	14–16 years
	Lateral epicondyle ⎭ humerus	11 years	13 years
	Upper end of radius	5 years	14–16 years
	Upper end of ulna	9 years	14–16 years
3. X-ray wrist AP view	Lower end of radius	2 years ⎫	16–18 years
	Lower end of ulna	6 years ⎭	
	Carpal bones:		
	Capitate	2nd month	
	Hamate	3rd month	
	Triquetrum	3rd year	
	Lunate	4th year	
	Scaphoid ⎫	5th year	
	Trapezium ⎭		
	Tra-pezoid	6th year	
	Pisiform	10–12 years	
	Base of 1st metacarpal	3rd year	15 years
	Phalanges	5–7 years	16–18 years
4. X-ray pelvis AP view	Upper end of femur:		
	Head	2 years ⎫	14–16
	Greater trochanter	5 years ⎬	years
	Lesser trochanter	12 years ⎭	
	Ischio-pubic ramus		Union 6th year
	Tri-radiate cartilage ⎫	Commences at	Completes at
	Ossification ⎭	13 years	15 years
	Iliac crest	14–16 years	18 years
	Ischial tuberosity	16–18 years	20–22 years
5. X-ray knee joint AP view	Lower end of femur	9th month IUL	
	Upper end of tibia	At birth ⎫	16–18 years
	Upper end of fibula	4th year ⎭	
6. X-ray ankle joint	Lower end of tibia ⎫	1st year	14–16 years
	Lower end of fibula ⎭		

EXERCISE

X-ray Shoulder Joint—AP View

Exercise 2.1

Table 2.2: X-ray shoulder joint—AP view

Name of ossification centre	Age of appearance	State of appearance	Age of fusion	State of fusion	Inference
1. Upper end of humerus					
(a) Head	1st year	after 5 years they all fuses together	16–18 years		
(b) Greater tubercle	2nd year				
(c) Lesser tubercle	5th year				
2. Acromion	14–16 years		18 years		
3. Coracoid process	3 years		16–18 years		

Opinion:

I am of the opinion that the above individual is aged above .... years and below .... years based on radiological examination.

Professor of Forensic Medicine
.... Medical college ....
Registration No. ....

X-ray Elbow Joint—AP View

Exercise 2.2

Table 2.3: X-ray elbow joint—AP view

Name of ossification centre	Age of appearance	State of appearance	Age of fusion	State of fusion	Inference
Capitulum	1 year		14–16 years		
Medial epicondyle	5–7 years		16 years		
Trochlea	9 years		14–16 years		
Lateral epicondyle	11 years		13 years		
Upper end of radius	5 years		14–16 years		
Upper end of ulna	9 years		14–16 years		

Opinion:

I am of the opinion that the above individual is aged above .... years and below .... years based on radiological examination.

Professor of Forensic Medicine
.... Medical college ....
Registration No. ....

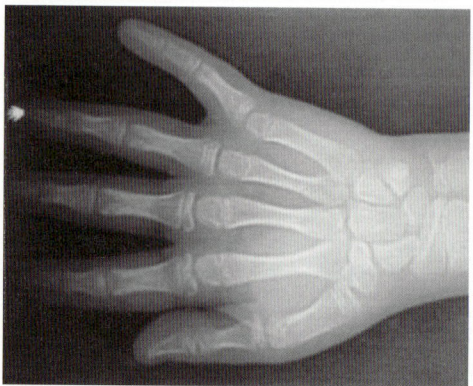

Fig. 2.4: X-ray wrist joint—AP view, pisiform not appeared, age is less than 12 years

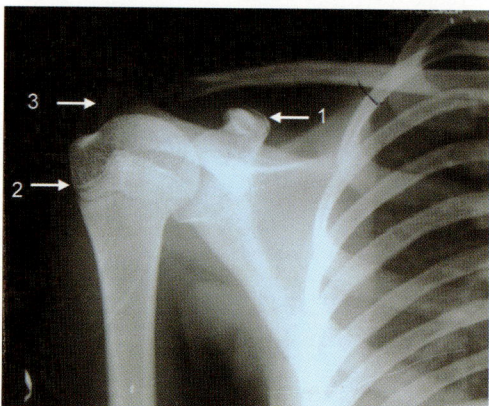

Fig. 2.5: X-ray shoulder joint (1) Ossification centre for coracoid process appeared (above 3 years) but not fused (below 18 years) (2) All the three ossification centres in the upper end of humerus appeared and fused with each other (above 6 years) but not with the shaft (below 18 years) (3) Ossification centre for acromion process appeared (above 14 years) but not fused (below 18 years)

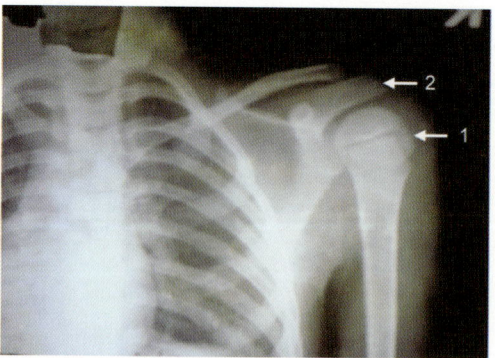

Fig. 2.6: X-ray shoulder joint (1) All the three ossification centres in the upper end of humerus appeared and fused with each other (above 6 years) but not with the shaft (below 18 years) (2) Ossification centre for acromion process not appeared (below 16 years)

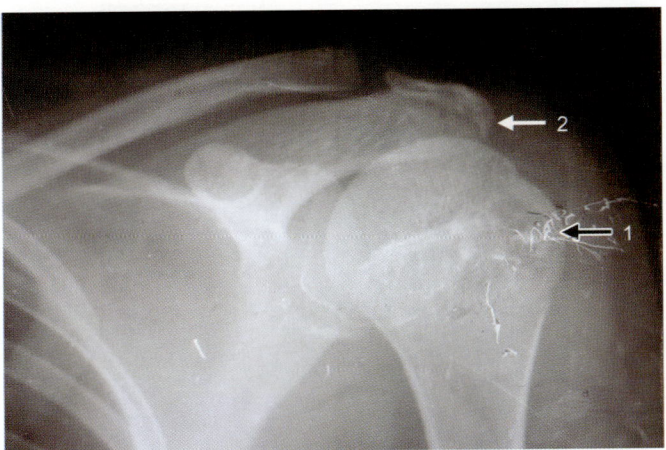

Fig. 2.7: X-ray shoulder joint (1) All the three ossification centres in the upper end of humerus appeared and fused with each other (above 6 years) but not with the shaft (below 18 years) (2) Ossification centre for acromion process appeared (above 14 years) but not fused (below 18 years)

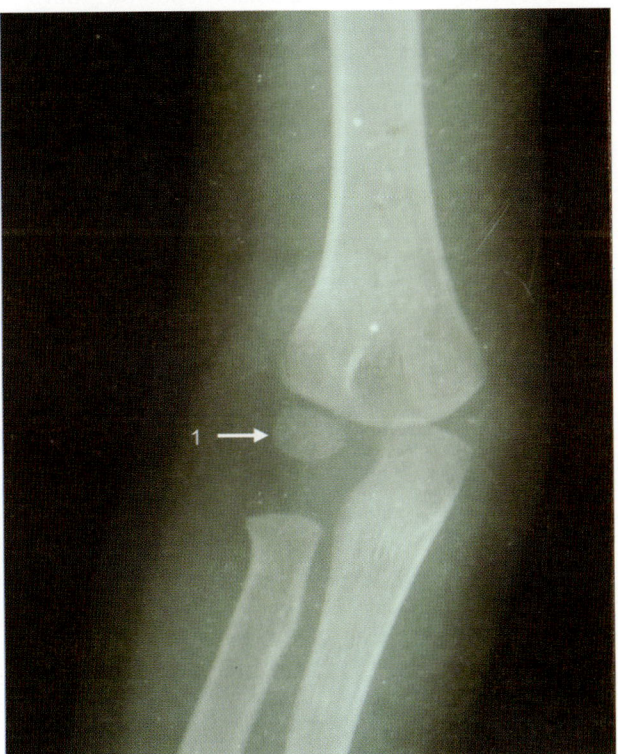

Fig. 2.8: X-ray elbow joint (AD view) (1) Ossification centre for capitulum appeared (above 1 year) but not fused (below 16 years). All the other centres around the elbow joint have not appeared (below 5 years)

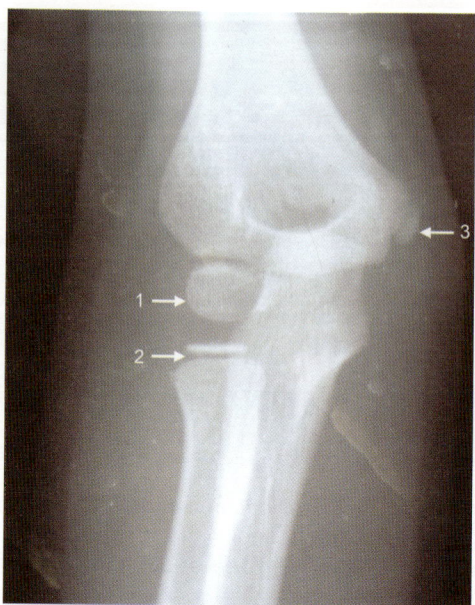

Fig. 2.9: X-ray elbow joint (1) Ossification centre for capitulum appeared (above 1 year) but not fused (below 16 years) (2) Ossification centre for upper end of radius appeared (above 5 years) but not fused (below 16 years) (3) Ossification centre for medial epicondyle appeared (above 5 years) but not fused (below 16 years)

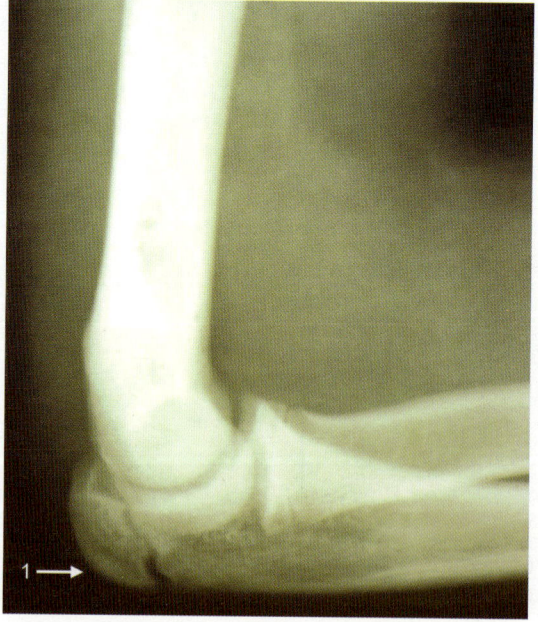

Fig. 2.10: X-ray elbow joint (lateral view) (1) Ossification centre for upper end of ulna appeared (above 9 years) but not fused (below 16 years)

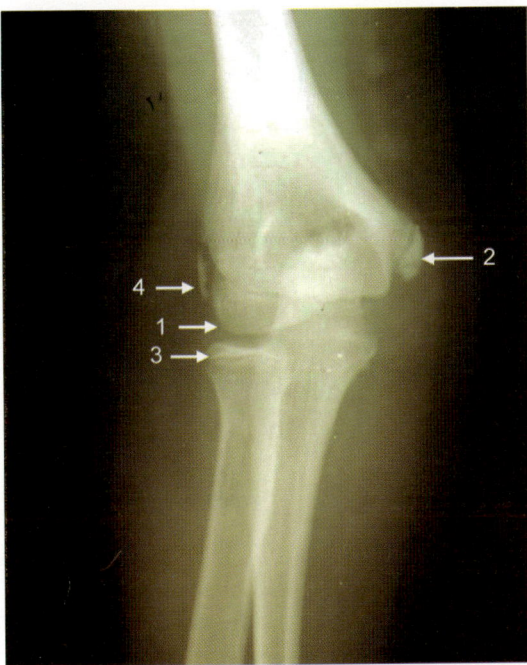

Fig. 2.11: X-ray elbow joint (1) Ossification centre for capitulum appeared (above 1 year) but not fused (below 16 years) (2) Ossification centre for upper end of radius appeared (above 5 years) but not fused (below 16 years) (3) Ossification centre for medial epicondyle appeared (above 5 years) but not fused (below 16 years) (4) Ossification centre for lateral epicondyle appeared (above 11 years) but not fused (below 13 years)

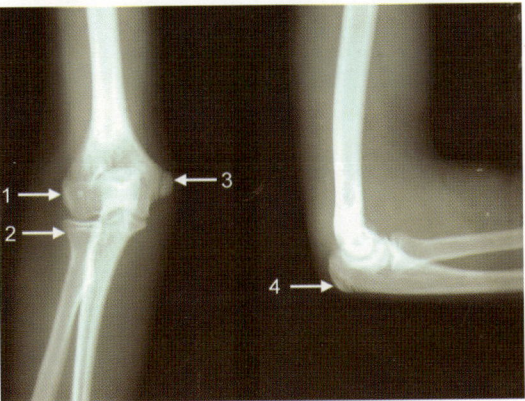

Fig. 2.12: X-ray elbow joint (AP and lateral view) (1) Ossification centre for capitulum fused (above 14 years) (2) Ossification centre for upper end of radius appeared (above 5 years) but not fused (below 16 years) (3) Ossification centre for medial epicondyle appeared (above 5 years) but not fused (below 16 years) (4) Ossification centre for upper end of ulna appeared (above 9 years) but not fused (below 16 years)

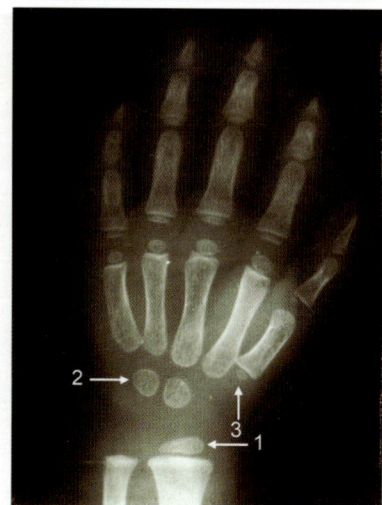

Fig. 2.13: X-ray wrist joint (1) Ossification centre for lower end of radius appeared (above 2 years) but not fused (below 18 years) (2) Only two carpal bones capitate (2 months) and hamate (3 months) have appeared (3) Ossification centre for base of 1st metacarpal has appeared (above 3 years) but not fused (below 15 years)

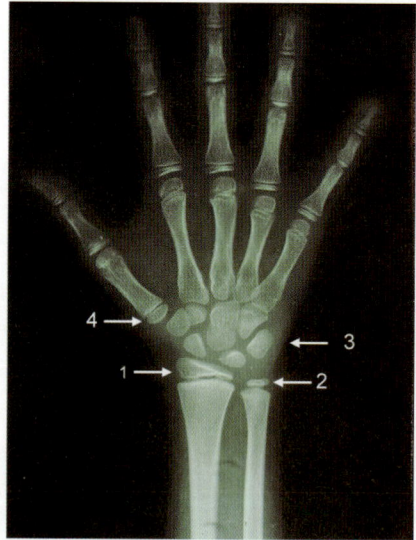

Fig. 2.14: X-ray wrist joint (1) Ossification centre for lower end of radius appeared (above 2 years) but not fused (below 18 years) (2) Ossification centre for lower end of ulna appeared (above 6 years) but not fused (below 18 years) (3) All the carpal bones except pisiform have appeared (below 12 years) (4) Ossification centre for base of 1st metacarpal has appeared (above 3 years) but not fused (below 15 years)

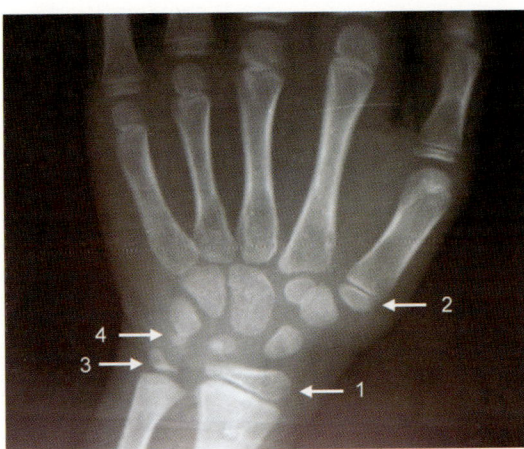

Fig. 2.15: X-ray wrist joint (1) Ossification centre for lower end of radius appeared (above 2 years) but not fused (below 18 years) (2) Ossification centre for base of 1st metacarpal has appeared (above 3 years) but not fused (below 15 years) (3) Ossification centre for lower end of ulna appeared (above 6 years) but not fused (below 18 years) (4) All the 8 carpal bones have appeared (above 10 years)

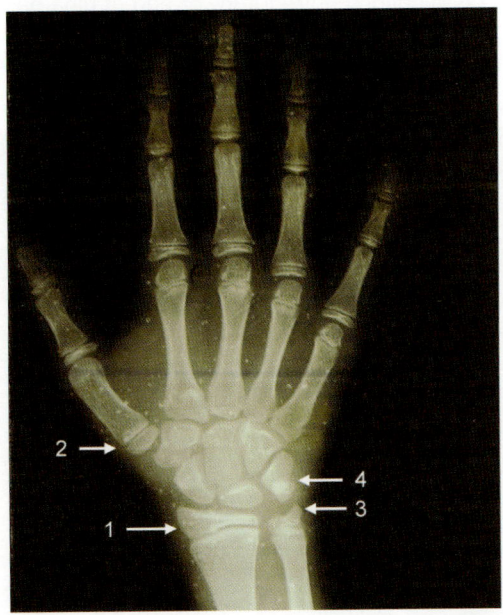

Fig. 2.16: X-ray wrist joint (1) Ossification centre for lower end of radius appeared (above 2 years) but not fused (below 18 years) (2) Ossification centre for base of 1st metacarpal has appeared (above 3 years) but not fused (below 15 years) (3) Ossification centre for lower end of ulna appeared (above 6 years) but not fused (below 18 years) (4) All the 8 carpal bones have appeared (above 10 years)

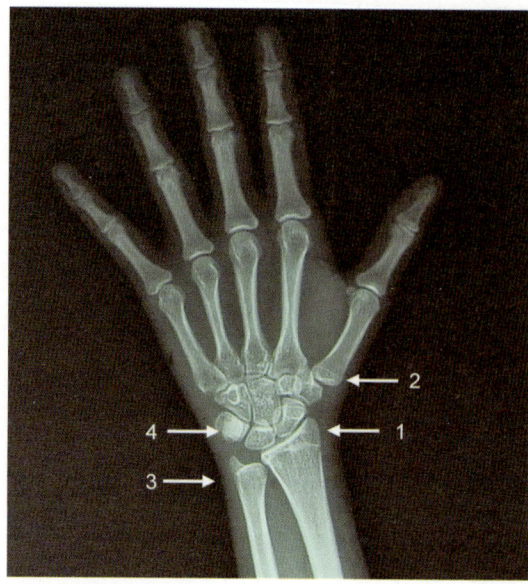

Fig. 2.17: X-ray wrist joint (1) Ossification centre for lower end of radius appeared (above 2 years) but not fused (below 18 years) (2) Ossification centre for base of 1st metacarpal has fused (above 15 years) (3) Ossification centre for lower end of ulna has fused (above 16 years) (4) All the 8 carpal bones have appeared (above 10 years)

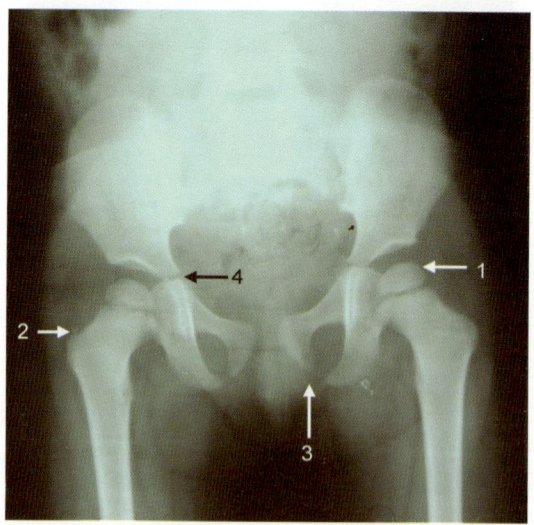

Fig. 2.18: X-ray pelvis (1) Ossification centre for head of femur appeared (above 2 years) but not fused (below 16 years) (2) Ossification centre for greater trochanter not appeared (below 5 years) (3) Ischio-pubic rami not united (below 6 years) (4) Tri-radiate cartilage not obliterated (below 15 years)

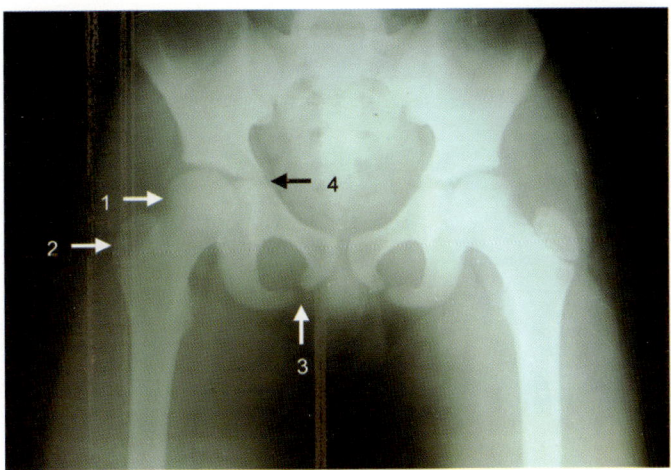

Fig. 2.19: X-ray pelvis (1) Ossification centre for head of femur appeared (above 2 years) but not fused (below 16 years) (2) Ossification centre for greater trochanter appeared (above 5 years) but not fused (below 16 years) (3) Ischio-pubic rami not united (below 6 years) (4) Tri-radiate cartilage not obliterated (below 15 years)

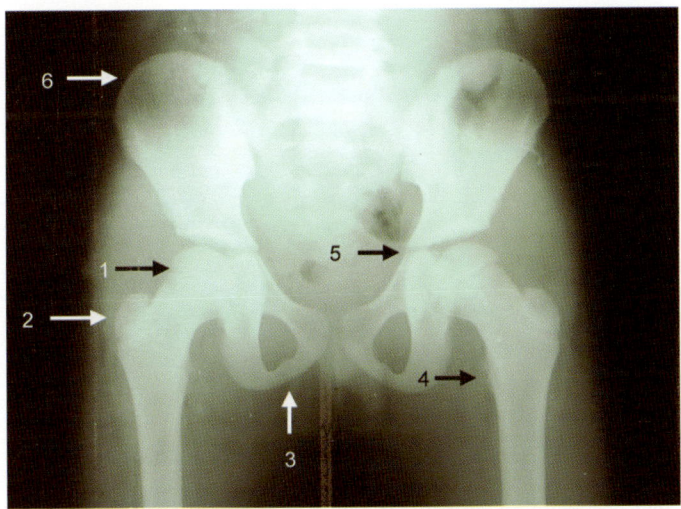

Fig. 2.20: X-ray pelvis (1) Ossification centre for head of femur appeared (above 2 years) but not fused (below 16 years) (2) Ossification centre for greater trochanter appeared (above 5 years) but not fused (below 16 years) (3) Ischio-pubic rami united (above 6 years) (4) Ossification centre for lesser trochanter not appeared (below 12 years) (5) Tri-radiate cartilage not obliterated (below 15 years) (6) Ossification centre for Iliac crest not appeared (below 14 years)

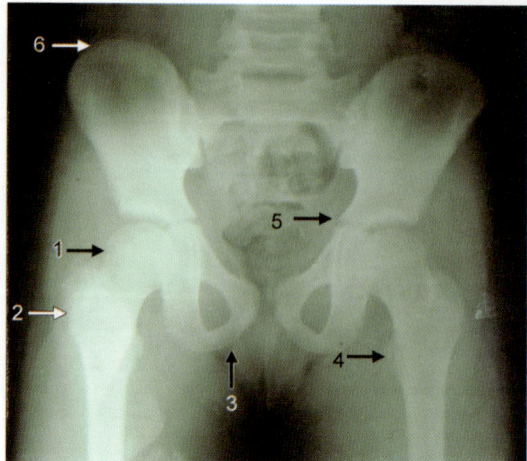

Fig. 2.21: X-ray pelvis (1) Ossification centre for head of femur appeared (above 2 years) but not fused (below 16 years) (2) Ossification centre for greater trochanter appeared (above 5 years) but not fused (below 16 years) (3) Ischio-pubic rami united (above 6 years) (4) Ossification centre for lesser trochanter appeared (above 12 years) but not fused (below 16 years) (5) Tri-radiate cartilage not obliterated (below 15 years) (6) Ossification centre for Iliac crest not appeared (below 14 years)

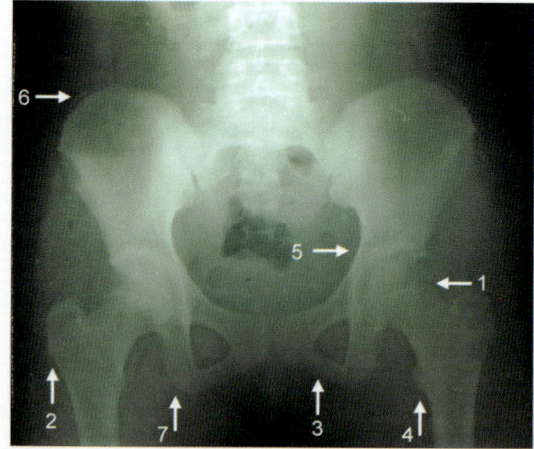

Fig. 2.22: X-ray pelvis (1) Ossification centre for head of femur fused (above 14 years) (2) Ossification centre for greater trochanter fused (above 14 years) (3) Ischio-pubic rami united (above 6 years) (4) Ossification centre for lesser trochanter fused (above 14 years) (5) Tri-radiate cartilage obliterated (above 13 years) (6) Ossification centre for Iliac crest just appeared (above 14 years) on the lateral sides (7) Ossification centre for ischial tuberosity not appeared (below 18 years)

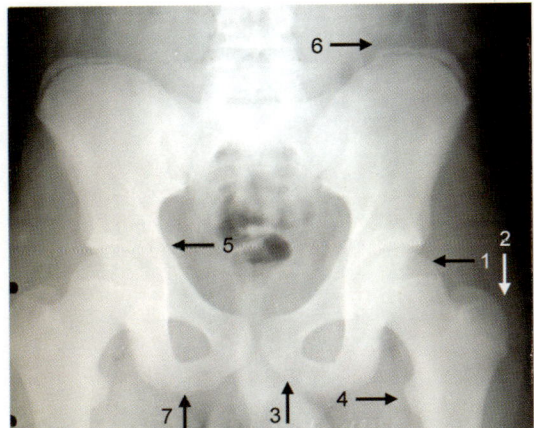

Fig. 2.23: X-ray pelvis (1) Ossification centre for head of femur fused (above 14 years) (2) Ossification centre for greater trochanter fused (above 14 years) (3) Ischio-pubic rami united (above 6 years) (4) Ossification centre for lesser trochanter fused (above 14 years) (5) Tri-radiate cartilage obliterated (above 13 years) (6) Ossification centre for Iliac crest appeared (above 16 years) but not fused (below 18 years) (7) Ossification centre for ischial tuberosity appeared (above 16 years) but not fused (below 20 years)

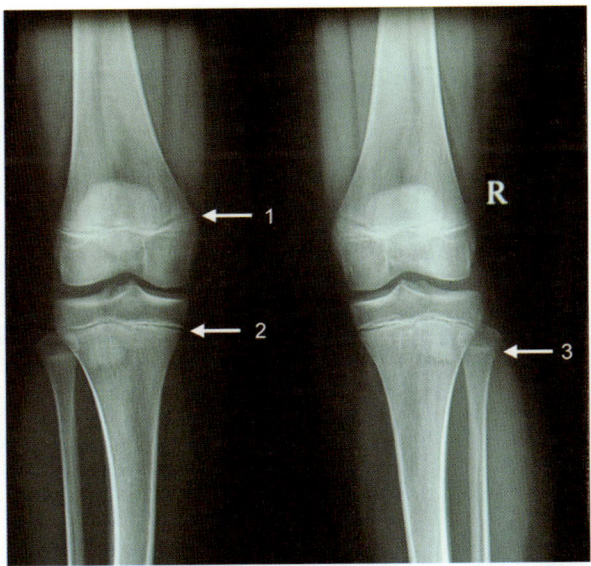

Fig. 2.24: X-ray knee joint (1) Ossification centre for lower end of femur appeared (above 9 months of IUL) but not fused (below 18 years) (2) Ossification centre for upper end of tibia appeared (above 10 months of IUL) but not fused (below 18 years) (3) Ossification centre for upper end of fibula appeared (above 4 years) but not fused (below 18 years)

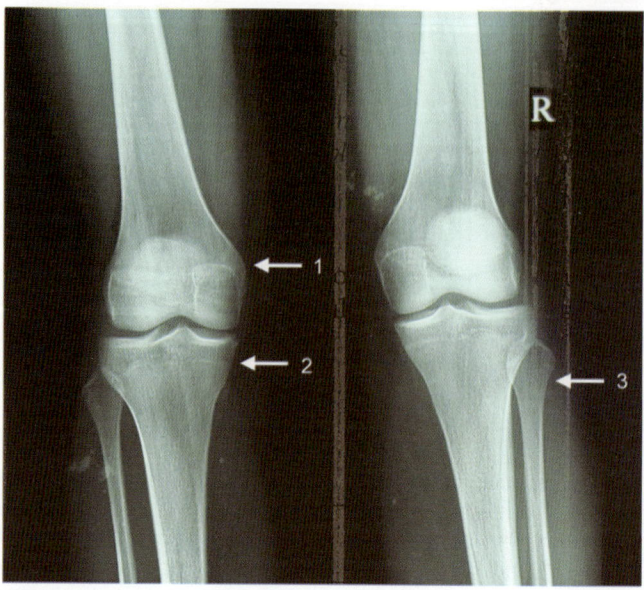

Fig. 2.25: X-ray knee joint (1) Ossification centre for lower end of femur fused (above 16 years) (2) Ossification centre for upper end of tibia fused (above 16 years) (3) Ossification centre for upper end of fibula fused (above 16 years)

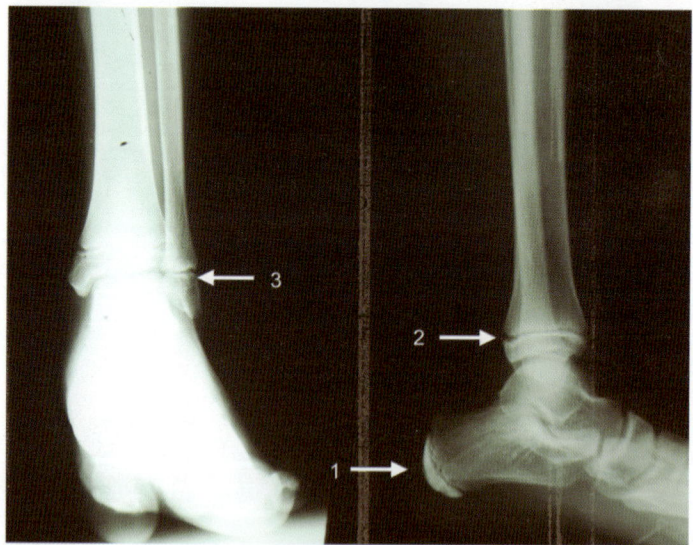

Fig. 2.26: X-ray ankle joint (1) Secondary Ossification centre for calcaneum appeared (above 6 years) but not fused (below 16 years) (2) Ossification centre for lower end of tibia appeared (above 1 year) but not fused (below 16 years) (3) Ossification centre for lower end of fibula appeared (above 1 year) but not fused (below 16 years)

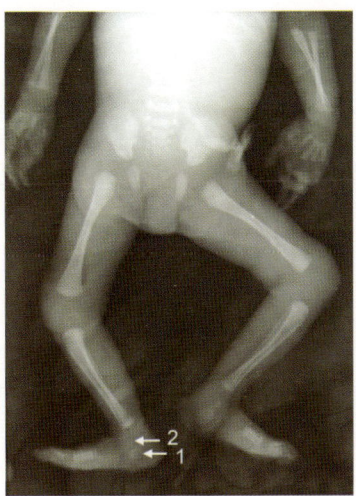

Fig. 2.27: X-ray foetus (1) Ossification centre for calcaneum appeared (above 6 months of IUL) (2) Ossification centre for talus appeared (above 7 months of IUL)

Exercise 2.3

Table 2.4: Wrist joint

Name of ossification centre	Age of appearance	State of appearance	Age of fusion	State of fusion	Inference
Lower end of radius	2 years ⎫		16–18 years		
Lower end of ulna	6 years ⎭				
Carpal bones:					
Capitate	2nd month				
Hamate	3rd month				
Triquetrum	3rd year				
Lunate	4th year				
Scaphoid	5th year				
Trapezium ⎫ Trapezoid ⎭	6th year				
Pisiform	10–12 years				
Base of 1st metacarpal	3rd year		15 years		
Phalanges	5–7 years		16–18 years		

Opinion:

I am of the opinion that the above individual is aged above .... years and below .... years based on radiological examination.

Professor of Forensic Medicine
.... Medical college ....
Registration No. ....

Exercise 2.4

Table 2.5: Pelvis

Name of ossification centre	Age of appearance	State of appearance	Age of fusion	State of fusion	Inference
Upper end of femur					
Head	2 years ⎱		14–16 years		
Greater trochanter	5 years ⎬				
Lesser trochanter	12 years ⎰				
Ischio-pubic ramus			Union 6th year		
Tri-radiate cartilage	Commences at		Completes at		
Ossification	13 years	⎱	15 years		
Iliac crest	14–16 years	⎰	18 years		
Ischial tuberosity	16–18 years		20–22 years		

Opinion:

I am of the opinion that the above individual is aged above .... years and below .... years based on radiological examination.

Professor of Forensic Medicine
...........Medical college ....
Registration No. ....

Register No. ....

Department of Forensic Medicine
Age Estimation Proforma

Requisition from The Judicial Magistrate of/Inspector of ....
vide letter/crime no. .... dated ....

1. Name of the individual   :
2. Sex   :
3. Parent's or guardian's name   :
4. Residential address   :
5. Occupation   :
6. Marital status   :
7. Age as alleged by
    (a) Individual to be examined   :
    (b) People or Police accompanying   :
8. Persons accompanying or brought by   :
9. Time, date and place of examination   :

10. Consent of the individual for examination   :
11. Signature of the individual consenting or his guardian   :
12. Marks of identification
    1.
    2.

Physical Examination

1. Height   :
2. Weight   :
3. Breadth   :
4. Chest girth at the level of the nipples   :
5. Abdominal girth at the level of the navel   :
6. General build and appearance   :
7. Voice   :   Infantile/Broken/Adult
8. Teeth   :   R————+————L
9. Hair   :
    Scalp
    Beard
    Moustache
    Axillary
    Pubic
10. Mammae—development   :
11. Generative organs—development   :
12. Date of menarche and regularity of cycle   :
13. Ossification   :
14. Opinion of age   :

Place: Professor of Forensic Medicine

Date: Register No. ....

Department of Forensic Medicine
Age Certificate

From the Physical, Dental and Radiological examination of .... S/o /D/o ....
.... resident of ....
.... bearing the identification marks.

1.
2.

I am of the opinion that the individual is aged above .... years and below .... years.

Place: Signature

Date:

MEDICOLEGAL IMPORTANCE OF AGE

Introduction

Age is an important factor in human life cycle and plays a vital role at every stage from conception till death of an individual. Even though registration of birth is made mandatory, the public response is still at low because of ignorance and illiteracy in our country. Age must be proved by documents not only in civil and criminal laws but also has importance in sports, marriage, contract, property, inheritance, etc. The best proof of age is the Birth Certificate and next is the School Leaving Certificate. Age recorded in the Voter ID, Ration Card and other cards issued by postal department, institutions and Employers are not the valid documentary proof for age. Hence in the absence of Birth Certificate and School Leaving Certificate the age must be ascertained by Medical examination with the most reliable age indicators. The age determined by a medical practitioner is not a conclusive proof of age; it is a mere opinion with a margin of error of two years on either side. Hence age determination is an important but a difficult task for a Registered Medical Practitioner; however, issuance of age certificate is a legal responsibility especially when it is sought from a court of law or an investigative authority.

To realize this important aspect a sound knowledge about applied aspects of age of human is essential for all doctors.

Importance of Age Before Birth

1. *Declaration of pregnancy:* Confirmation of pregnancy should be done 7 to 10 days after fertilization since the fertilized ovum should be implanted in the uterus. Premature declaration will invite embarrassment for the anxious couple as well as the doctor since there is every possibility of spontaneous expulsion without proper implantation.

2. *Embryonic phase:* Up to the 2nd month or 8 weeks it is called embryo since it does not look like human.

3. *Foetal stage:* From 3rd month or 12th week onwards it looks like a human and it is called Foetus. According to Medical Termination of Pregnancy Act 1971 a pregnancy can be terminated with strong indication by a single doctor. If the termination is carried out without any indications, neither with good intention nor for the benefit of the pregnant woman it is considered as illegal or criminal abortion. According to Section 312 IPC the Perpetrator of Criminal Abortion can be prosecuted and imprisoned up to 3 years.

4. *Quickening:* During 4th month or 16th week of pregnancy centres for bones appeared for almost all the bones and the foetus can move inside the uterus and the mother can feel the foetal movement. First perception of foetal movement by its mother is called Quickening. Normally the criminal abortion is punishable up to 3 years according to Section 312 IPC but abortion performed after quickening, the punishment is enhanced to 7 years.

5. 5th month or 20th week of pregnancy is the maximum allowable period for Medical Termination according to MTP Act 1971. It is to be carried out by two doctors. This restriction is relaxed on emergency conditions where the termination can be carried out by a single doctor with good intention of saving the life of the woman. Causing miscarriage without woman's consent attracts punishment up to 10 years of imprisonment according to Section 313 IPC.

6. *Medical viability:* A foetus of 6 months or 24 weeks is considered as matured enough to lead independent life if delivered with Intensive Neonatal Care sufficiently. Death of the woman caused by an act done with intent to cause miscarriage is punishable up to 10 years according to Section 314 IPC and if without consent life imprisonment is awarded.

7. *Legal viability:* Law considered that a foetus of 7 lunar months or 28 weeks old is capable of having an independent life in the event of expulsion from the womb. According to Section 315 IPC act done with intent to prevent child being born alive or to cause it to die after birth is punishable up to 10 years of imprisonment. Here the viability attainment has to be proved.

8. *Stillbirth:* A child born after attainment of viability (28 weeks) did not breath or show any other signs of life at any time after being completely born. As per the Indian Birth and Death Registration Act all cases of stillbirth should be registered properly.

9. *Full term:* 10 lunar months or 40 weeks is considered as normal period of pregnancy with little overlapping. According to Section 316 IPC whoever causes death of a quick unborn child is amounting to culpable homicide and can be punished up to 10 years imprisonment.

Importance of Age After Birth

1. *Infanticide:* Unlawful killing of a child under one year is known as infanticide which is dealt under Section 300 IPC. Murder can be punished under Section 302 IPC. In some countries like Canada, Australia and the UK killing of a child under one year of age by its mother is not murder since it could be due to postpartum depression (baby blues), hence the punishment is less.

2. *Concealment of birth:* According to Section 318 IPC concealment of birth by secret disposal of dead body of child whether the child died before or during or after birth is punishable with imprisonment up to 2 years.

3. 5 years: According to Hindu Minority and Guardianship Act 1956 a child under 5 years shall be in the custody of its mother. This is normal age for admission in school.

4. 7 years: According to Section 82 of IPC a child less than 7 years is not held responsible for his act.

5. 10 years: According to Section 369 IPC kidnapping or abducting a child less than 10 years with an intention of taking dishonestly any movable property shall be punished with imprisonment up to seven years.

6. 12 years:
   1. According to Section 83 IPC an offence committed by a child above 7 years and under 12 years is not held responsible, provided that the child is not attained sufficient mental maturity to understand the nature and consequences of his conduct on that occasion.
   2. According to Section 90 IPC consent given by a child under 12 years is not valid to undergo an act which is done in good faith and for benefit of the child.
   3. According to Section 89 IPC there is a remedy for the invalid consent explained under Section 90 IPC, consent can be given either by parent or guardian on behalf of the under 12 years child for an act which is done in good faith for the benefit of the child.

4. According to Section 317 of IPC exposure or Abandonment of a child less than 12 years of age by parents or any person having care shall be punished with imprisonment of 7 years.

5. According to Section 376 of IPC sexual intercourse by a man with his own wife whose age is below 12 years, he can be punished for rape with imprisonment up to 7–10 years but if her age is above 12 years but below 15 years he can be imprisoned up to 2 years only.

6. According to Indian Oath Amendment Act 1939, a child less than 12 years of age is exempted from taking oath.

7. According to Child Labour Act, a child under 12 years of age should not be engaged as a servent in shops and is punishable with 2 years imprisonment or fine of Rs. 20,000.

7. 14 years:

1. According to Indian Factory Act, a person below 14 years of age should not be employed in any factory or mine or in hazardous employment.

2. According to Indian Factory Act a person above 14 years but not below 15 years can be employed in a factory with conditions of not working continuously for more than 8 hours and no night duty.

8. 15 years:

1. According to Section 375 IPC sexual intercourse by a man with his own wife whose age is above 12 years but below 15 years is punishable up to two years imprisonment and if she is above 15 years, it is not an offence.

2. According to Indian Factory Act, a person of 15 years can be employed in a factory.

3. According to Section 160 of Criminal Procedure Code a police officer cannot compel a male below 15 years or any woman to appear before him at any place other than the place where such male or woman resides.

4. If a person of 15 years of age has committed the offence of murder, the police must record his age as 15 and he should be produce before the Juvenile Justice Board within 24 hours of his arrest. In case of doubt the Juvenile Justice Board will conduct an inquiry to ascertain the age by procuring documentary proof of age. In the absence of such documentary proof that person should be sent for medical examination to ascertain age according to Section 49 of Juvenile Justice Act 2000.

5. A wife may divorce her husband if the marriage was solemnized before attaining 15 years and repudiated the marriage after attaining the age of 15 years but before attaining 18 years as the Hindu Marriage Act 1955.

9. 16 years:

1. Age 16 is the age of consent for sexual intercourse in females, hence sexual intercourse with a girl below 16 years is amounting to rape even with her consent as per Section 375 of IPC and it is called Statutory Rape.

2. According to Section 363 A of IPC kidnapping or maiming a minor for purpose of begging is punishable with imprisonment of ten years for kidnapping and life

imprisonment for maiming. Under this section the age of a male person is 16 years and that of a girl is 18 years.

3. According to Indian Arms Act 1959 a person below the age of 16 years cannot keep any fire arm or ammunition in his possession.

10. 18 years: This is the age of majority since there is drastic change of an adolescent into adult. It has got a lot of legal bearings such as civil, criminal, social, medical, etc as follows.

1. *Criminal responsibility:* A juvenile is a person who has not completed 18 years of age. According to Juvenile Justice Act 1986, the discrimination of age between a boy and a girl was two years, i.e. a boy under 16 and a girl under 18 have been repealed by Section 2(K) of Juvenile Justice Act 2000 with retrospective effect. According to this Act any person between 12 and 18 years who have committed an offence is criminally responsible but are not to be treated as an adult person (i.e. above 18 years) and should be dealt under Juvenile Legislation and neither death sentence or life imprisonment should be imposed.

2. *Kidnapping:* According to Section 363 A of IPC kidnapping or maiming a minor in order to employment or begging shall be punishable with imprisonment up to 10 years and with maiming can be punished with imprisonment for life. This section discriminate a boy under 16 years as minor, whereas a girl under 18 years of age.

3. According to Section 366A of IPC whoever induces any girl under 18 years to go from any place by whatever means knowingly that she will be forced or seduced to illicit intercourse with another person is punishable up to 10 years imprisonment.

4. According to Sections 372 and 373 of IPC whoever sells or lets to hire or otherwise disposes (372) and whoever buys, hires or otherwise obtained possession (373) of any female under the age of 18 years for purposes of prostitution shall be punished with imprisonment up to 10 years.

5. According to Section 300 of IPC under exception 5, culpable homicide is not murder when the person whose death is caused being above the age of 18 years suffers death or takes the risk of death with his own consent.

6. According to Section 305 of IPC if any person under 18 years of age (any insane or any debrious person, any idiot or any person in a state of intoxication) commits suicide, whoever abets the commission of such suicide shall be punished with death or imprisonment for life or for a term not exceeding 10 years imprisonment.

7. According to Section 87 of IPC nothing is an offence by an act which is not intended or not known to cause death or grievous hurt to any such person of above 18 years who has given consent to face the risk of death or hurt. If the person is below 18 years his consent becomes invalid.

8. *Age and Medical practice:* According to Section 88 of IPC the ingredient is the same as that of 87 IPC but this is concerned with Medical Practice where the act is done in good faith and for the benefit of the individual. Hence any individual who is above 18 years of age can give consent to undergo surgery of any kind and any other diagnostic or therapeutic procedures which are having inherent risks of causing death or grievous hurt.

9. *Age and Medical practice:* According to Section 3(4) (a) of MTP Act 1971, a pregnant woman under 18 years cannot give consent for termination of her pregnancy, hence husband or guardian should give consent in written.

10. According to Section 2(F) of the Transplantation of Human Organs Act 1994 a person of above 18 years only can donate one of his/her paired organ for transplantation.

11. This is the age of voting in India

12. This is the age of marriage for girls.

13. This is the age for obtaining license to drive motorized vehicle.

14. This is the age for opening an independent account in any bank.

15. 18 years is the minimum age for entering into any type of contract.

16. Person of age 18 years and above only can make a valid will.

11. **20 years:**
    1. According to Section 293 of IPC whoever sells lets to hire, distributes, circulates or exhibits obscene objects to any person below the age of 20 years shall be punished with imprisonment of 3 years and Rs 2000 fine on first time and in the event of second or subsequent conviction with imprisonment of 7 years and Rs 5000 fine.
    2. According to Section 44 of the Juvenile Justice Act 2000, age 20 is the maximum age for a juvenile to stay in Care and Rehabilitation Center and on completion of 20 years he must be shifted to prison.

12. **21 years:**
    1. According to Section 366B of IPC whoever imports into India from any country outside India or from the state of Jammu and Kashmir any girl under 21 years for the purpose of illicit sexual intercourse shall be punished with imprisonment of 10 years.
    2. According to Section 5 (III) of the Hindu Marriage Act 1955, this is the age of marriage for male and marriage before attaining 21 years invites simple imprisonment of 15 days or Rs 1000 as fine or with both.

13. **25 years:** According to Article 84 (b) and Article 173 (b) of the Constitution of India, age 25 is the minimum age eligible to contest for membership of parliament and membership legislative assembly of state respectively.

14. **30 years:** According to the Article 84 (b) and 173 (b) of the Constitution of India, 30 years is the minimum age to contest for membership of Rajya Sabha and State Legislative Council.

15. **35 years:**
    1. 35 years of age is the minimum age for contesting in the election for the post of Vice President and President of India.
    2. 35 years of age is the minimum age for appointment of Governor to any state of India.

16. **40 years:** In Artificial Insemination donor, the age of the donor should not be above 40 years.

17. **45 to 50 years:** Normally a woman attains menopause between 45 and 50 years.

18. 55 to 65 years: This is the age of retirement from Government service. This age of retirement varies in Central Service and varies in different states ranging from 55 to 65 years.

    1. To charge an offence of infanticide, the age of the mother should be below the age of menopause.
    2. According to Section 416 of Criminal Procedure Code, if a woman sentenced to death is found to be pregnant, the death sentence awarded can be postponed up to 6 months after delivery or it may be altered to life imprisonment.
    3. A man is said to be potent and fertile till death but usually after 70–80 years the reproductivity gradually recedes.

3

Injury Examination and Wound Certificate

INTRODUCTION

Trauma has always been part of human life causing serious threat or disability with dependence due to various types of incidents like assault or accident resulting in various types of wound.

A *wound* is defined as any damage to any part of the body due to deliberate or accidental application of force.

The responsibility of doctors in dealing with injured victims falls in two categories.

1. Therapeutic responsibility involving alleviation of pain and suffering; prevention of immediate and delayed damages and promotion of quick recovery.
2. Legal responsibility where many doctors experience difficulties. However, it is the bounden duty of a doctor to assist the investigation for appropriate legal interpretation leading to a better judicial outcome. This can be done with a sound forensic knowledge so that the wounds can be appropriately assessed and properly documented. On many occasions the doctors are appreciated by the patient and others for their immediate, skillful clinical management but the lacunae in legal responsibility is exposed several weeks or months later, in a court of law when the documents are scrutinized and testified. To avoid this embarrassment in a court of law, a basic knowledge in forensic wound assessment is essential for all doctors.

The ultimate aim of examination of the victim (the assailant sometimes) is to reconstruct the events and circumstances that are responsible for the victim to sustain injuries.

ACCIDENT REGISTER

What is an Accident Register?

The accident register is a medicolegal document meant for documenting the relevant facts and physical findings on victims of violence by the CMO/EMO. The register is available in the casualty department of all hospitals.

What are the Cases to be Entered in the Accident Register?

The following cases pertaining to:

- Victims of attempted suicide or parasuicide
- Victims of unlawful or illegal acts

- Victims of all types of accidents
- Victims of animal bite, snake bite or insect stings, etc.
- Assailant who also sustained injuries in assault cases.
- All cases of unexplained coma
- All cases of poisoning
- All cases of brought dead/death on arrival

METHOD OF MAKING AN ENTRY IN THE ACCIDENT REGISTER

As with any other medicolegal document the accident register also comprises three parts.

1. Preamble
2. Body
3. Conclusion

Preamble

The following data should be entered.

- Serial number
- Time, date and place of examination
- Personal data of the patient (including two identification marks such as moles/tattoo marks/scar) on the visible part of the body.
- Brief details of the person who brought in/accompanying the victim. If brought by police officer, memo number, name of the police station, rank of the police officer who is investigating, number name and rank of the police constable/or if by others their name, state of relationship to the victim.
- Consent: Many a time the serious nature of the injury/condition of the patient does not require consent (Implied) but in cases of fabricated injuries or falsifying history, consent may be helpful to avoid the possibility of litigation against the doctor, at a later date.

The preamble is useful in establishing the positive identification of the victim at the time of trial at a later date.

Body

Body of the accident register is concerned with the factual findings on clinical examination. This begins with recording the history of the event briefly, as is narrated by the victim. If the victim is not in a position to depose, due to disturbance of consciousness, physical or mental distress, the relative or any other person who was with the victim at the time of the alleged event can explain. This history of event should cover 5 W s

1. When: Time, day and date
2. Where: Place of occurrence
3. Why: Motive of the event either intentional or accidental
4. By Whom: Known or unknown person, one or more than one individual
5. With What: Type of weapon, or vehicle or any other means.

After listening carefully and being convinced, the history should be written legibly without overwriting or rewriting.

Examination Under Two Headings

i. General Examination

Physical characters such as height, weight, circumferences of chest and abdomen, etc along with vital parameters such as pulse, blood pressure, respiratory rate, state of consciousness, pupillary size and reaction to light, accommodation of both eyes and abnormal odour in breath (alcohol) should be noted. This examination also includes conventional screening examination for cardiovascular system, respiratory system and locomotor system. If any abnormality is detected in any of these systems, the person must be referred to the concerned specialist for opinion, especially whether an injury is the effect of the alleged event or is preexisting and detected incidentally. If there is a smell of alcohol perceived in the breath, concurrent examination of drunkenness also should be carried out after getting informed written consent of the victim along with collection of blood and urine. If the victim is in a state of coma, find out the cause of coma clinically, whether due to assault, alcohol or other disorders or drugs and treatment should be prioritized by the concerned specialists.

ii. Specific Examination

It involves the examination of the wound/wounds for clinical assessment corroborating with the events, and circumstances deposed by the victim.

To document a wound, first the type of the wound (morphological type — abrasion, contusion, laceration, deformity with swelling, incised wound, chop wound, penetrating wound or perforating wound) must be identified. Second, the location on the body (anatomical site) must be specified in relation to anatomical landmarks. Third, the dimensions of the wound— two dimensions in abrasions and contusions, three dimensions in lacerations and incised wounds (depth not necessary to measure but in relation to the structure of tissues exposed in the floor of the wound, e.g. skin deep, muscle deep or bone deep) and in punctured wounds, never probe the wound in the living person. Fourth, the state of the wound in relation to the time elapsed after sustaining such as colour, swelling and discharge of blood, serous or purulent fluid will reflect the age of the wound. Lastly, corroborate the wound with the alleged weapon used and the circumstances of the alleged assault/accident.

Conclusion

The concluding part of the document should contain the opinion by corroborating with the alleged history and the observed findings as:

1. The alleged time and manner (regarding the nature of weapon, time of assault) is consistent or inconsistent with the clinical findings.
2. Intimation to the police is required/not required.
3. Dying declaration is required/not required.
4. The clinical opinion regarding the severity of injury is simple/grievous. In case of multiple injuries indicate the category to which each injury belongs.

OBJECTIVES OF WOUND ASSESSMENT

Medical:
1. To relieve pain and suffering
2. To repair the damage
3. To prevent infection/complications
4. To revive and restore health
5. To prevent defect/deformity
6. To assess the degree of disability
7. To offer clinical opinion

Legal:
1. To corroborate the history
    (a) To assess the nature of weapon
    (b) To assess the number of assailants
    (c) To assess the time of assault/accident
2. To assess the nature and severity
3. To reconstruct the events
4. To retrieve trace evidences if present
5. To assess the stage of healing in delayed reporting
6. To document the injuries
7. To initiate legal action
8. To appraise in the criminal court during trial

Principles

The accident register should be written in triplicate. It should be duly signed only by the casualty doctor in his/her own handwriting. The original should be sent to the jurisdiction magistrate court, the duplicate should be given to the police and the triplicate should be retained for future reference.

1. Injured victim should be immediately attended.
2. Examination should not be refused for want of police referral memo.
3. Treatment should not be withheld for want of money.
4. No consent is required in life threatening injuries.
5. Informed refusal/against medical advice should be documented and the same must be signed by the victim and or accompanying relative.
6. Preventive and prophylactic treatment should be administered even on refusal/against medical advice/referral cases. General condition should be stabilized before shifting to another hospital.
7. Entry in the accident register is mandatory in all cases even in refusal of admission/ against medical advice
8. Intimation to the police is essential in all cases of assault.
9. Arrange to record the dying declaration in seriously injured victim of assault.
10. Record the statement in presence of two uninterested witnesses, in cases of impending death/delay in arrival of Magistrate.

Procedure

Preliminary Data

(a) Time, date and place of examination

(b) Name, age, sex, address and occupation of the victim.

(c) Name, number and rank of the police personnel who brought the victim, with the crime no. and station to which he is attached.

or

Name and his relationship to the patient if accompanied by person other than a police constable.

(d) Two identification marks preferably on exposed parts of the body

(e) Though consent is not required (implied), in cases of custodial torture, or contradictory or unconvincing history, written consent should be obtained.

(f) Remarks about police intimation/dying declaration.

History Evaluation

Allow the victim to narrate the circumstances and surroundings of the incident and clarify regarding the five important W s.

1. Who has assaulted or caused accident, known or unknown (never mention the name of the person, since the doctor does not know that person)?

2. When did the assault/accident occur?

3. Where did it occur?

4. Why did it occur?

5. What kind of weapon/vehicle used?

General Examination

(a) Evaluate the history of the event and document it.

(b) Record vital parameters such as

- Higher functions : State of consciousness, orientation to time and space, speech and memory for recent and remote events.
- Cardiovascular : Pulse, BP, heart sounds
- Respiratory : Rate of respiration, breath sounds, abnormal breath sounds.
- Abdomen : Pain, tenderness, guarding, rigidity, organomegaly, bowel sounds.
- Ocular : State of the eyelids and corneal reflex. Pupillary size, reaction to light and accommodation. Color of conjunctiva.
- Oral cavity : Lips, gum, teeth, tongue, salivation, bleeding and odour in the breath.

Specific Examination

Injuries:
    (a) Type
    (b) Size
    (c) Site
    (d) Surface
    (e) Stage of healing
    (f) Number of injuries
    (g) Consistency with alleged weapon, time and manner
    (h) Nature of injuries whether simple, grievous, etc

Investigation

To Rule Out:

1. Bony lesions or foreign body (broken weapon) with X-rays.
2. Intracranial lesion with X-ray and CT scan
3. Intra-abdominal lesion with USG abdomen

If there is severe blood loss—preliminary investigation for blood transfusion to be done in consultation with concerned specialist by calling them to casualty.

Treatment Given

Injection tetanus toxoid—1 ampoule IM

Wound suture, debridement and dressing

Analgesic, antibiotic

Advised admission or to attend OP.

All the above details are properly recorded in triplicate in the accident register with signature of the CMO/EMO with date.

1. The original is sent to the court
2. Duplicate to the police
3. Triplicate for reference and to be used while giving evidence in court

Importance of an Accident Register

1. It is the documentary evidence of an unlawful act recorded by a competent doctor.
2. It is the preliminary document for the investigator to initiate action against the assailants.
3. It is the vital document to claim compensation from the Accident Claims Tribunal.
4. It is an important corroborative evidence in the event of death.
5. It is the preliminary document for issuing a wound certificate.
6. It is a proof of medical treatment, during an emergency.

Accident Register

Date: .... Time: .... Sl. No: ....

Hospital Name: .... Hospital No: ....

Name: .... Age: .... Sex: ....

Address: .... Occupation: ....

Married/single: ....

Brought by: ....

Identification Marks:

      1.

      2.

Consent: Written consent obtained

History of the alleged event by patient/relative:

Past and personal history:

Medical History:

Not a diabetic/hypertensive/ischemic heart disease.

General Examination

General condition fair, conscious, oriented

                    Pulse—   BP—

CVS

RS

CNS

Abdomen

Intimation to the police: Yes/ No

Dying declaration: Necessary/Not necessary

Local Examination

List of Injuries:

1.

2.

3.

Investigation:

                → AP view

X-ray

                ↘ Lateral view

Treatment:

- Injection TT 0.5 ml given intramuscular
- Wound suturing done
- Analgesics and antibiotics given

Advice:

Date:

                                    Signature of Medical Officer

                                      Registration No....................

Place:

WOUND CERTIFICATE

Definition

It is a medicolegal document issued by the doctor who has examined the injured victim and entered the details in the accident register.

Significance

1. It is a conciscd report reproduced from the accident register.
2. It is a proof of physical violence.
3. It is the basis to initiate criminal action against the assailant.
4. It is the basis for penalizing the accused by a court after oral testimony.
5. It is an important document to claim compensation through Motor Accident Claims Tribunal Court.
6. It is the basis to get a disability certificate.

Wound Certificate

WC.NO:
AR.NO:
HOSPITAL NO:

Certified that I, Dr .... have examined (Name) ...., (S/o or D/o)
........................, (Age) ...., (Sex) ...., residing at (Address) ....,
on (Date) .... at (Time) .... he/she was identified with (identification marks)

1.
2.

The following injuries were found on his body.

S. No	Type (cm)	Size	Site	Stage of healing/age of the wound	Type of force/weapon	Remarks simple/grievous
1.						
2.						
3.						

Opinion:

I am of the opinion based on clinical findings that injuries no. 1 and 2 are simple and injury no. 3 is grievous. The examination findings are consistent/inconsistent with alleged history and the time and manner stated.

Signature of the Medical Officer
Registration No.....................

Date:
Place:

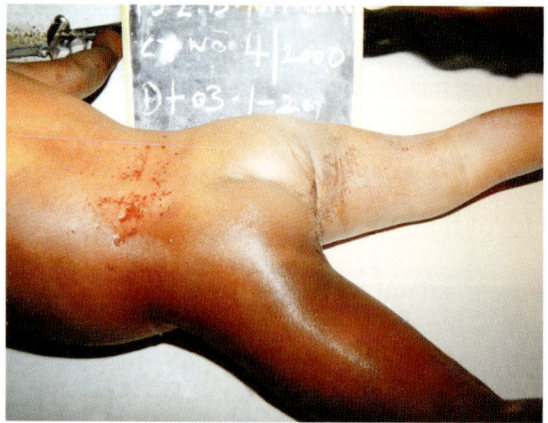

Fig. 3.1: Punctate abrasion

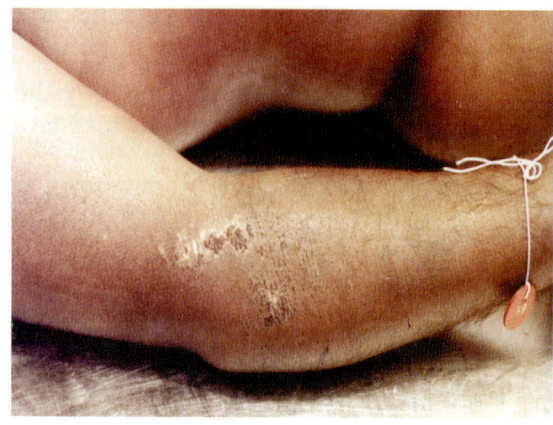

Fig. 3.2: Healing abrasion

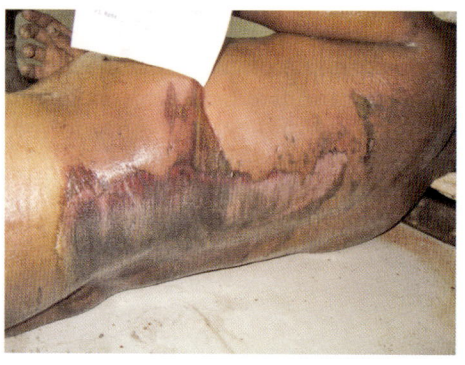

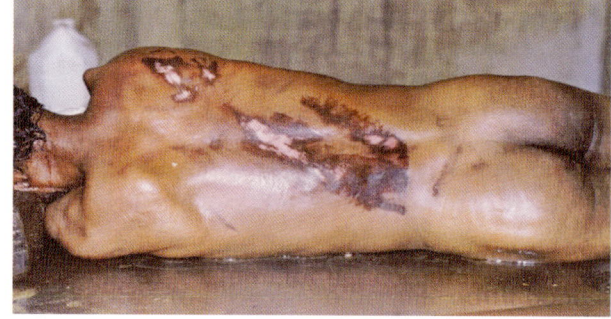

Fig. 3.3: Graze abrasion

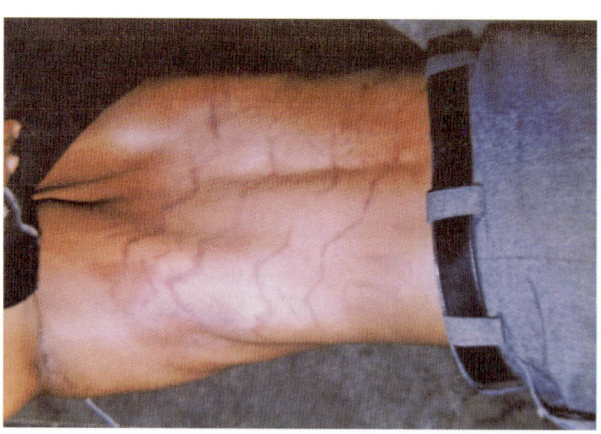

Fig. 3.4: Patterned abrasion (tyre tread)

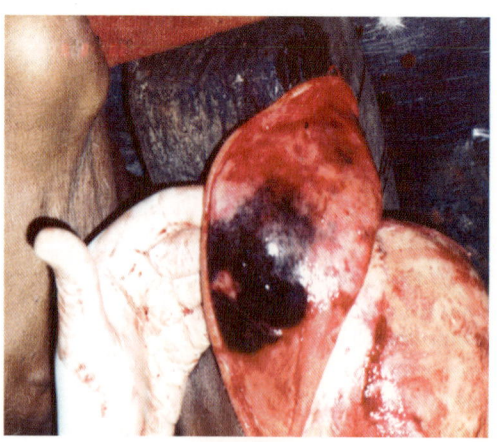

Fig. 3.5: Contusion

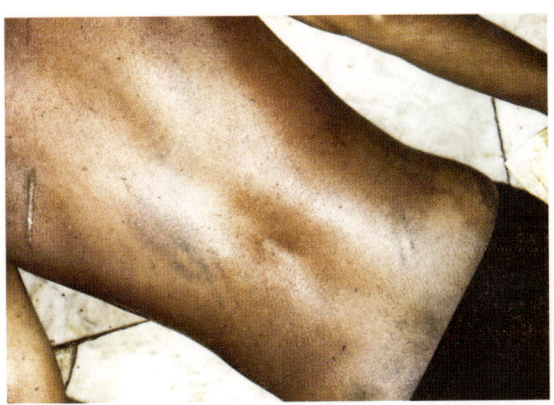

Fig. 3.6: Patterned contusion (tramline)

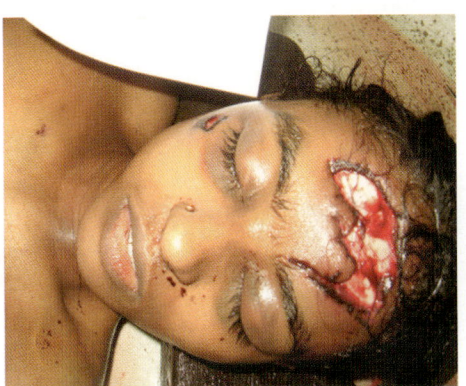

Fig. 3.7: Laceration

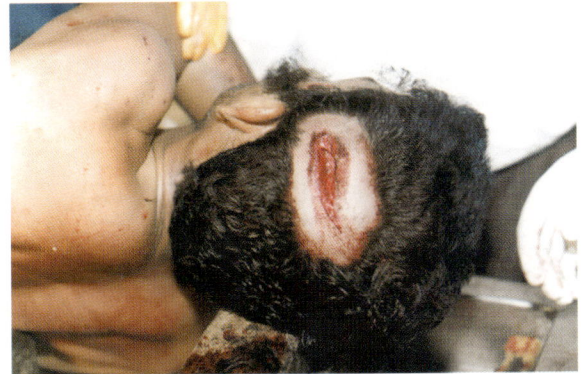

Fig. 3.8: Split (incised looking) laceration

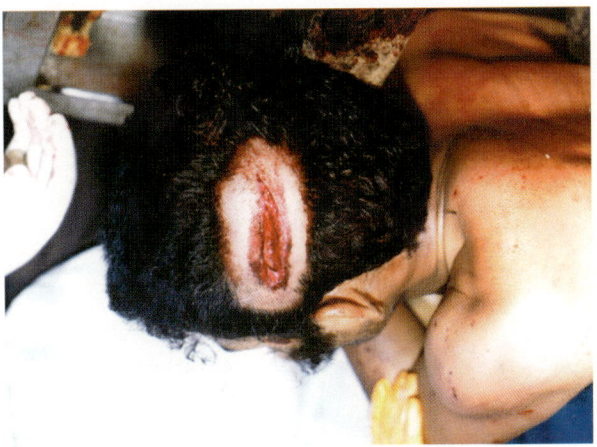

Fig. 3.9: Laceration with marginal abrasion

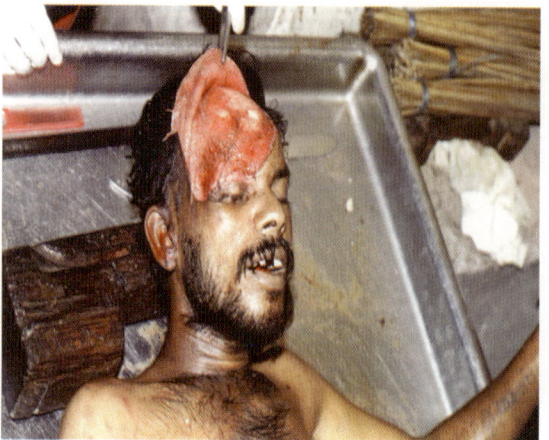

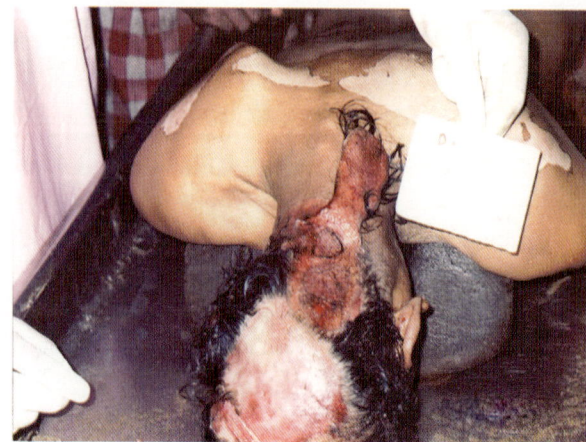

Fig. 3.10: Avulsion laceration

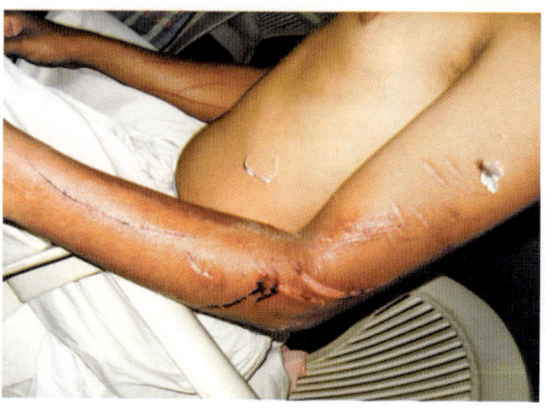

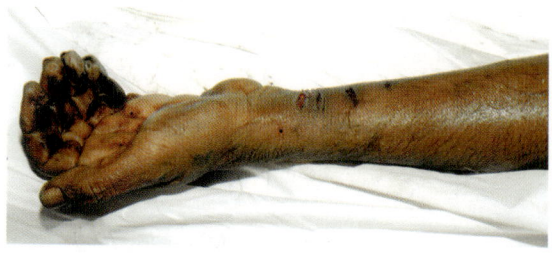

Fig. 3.11: Incised wound

Fig. 3.12: Self-inflicted incised wounds

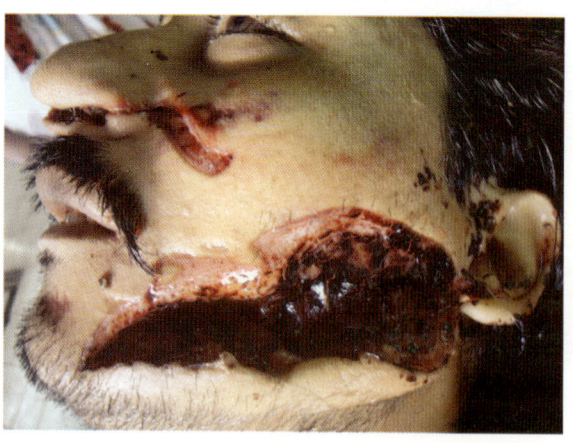

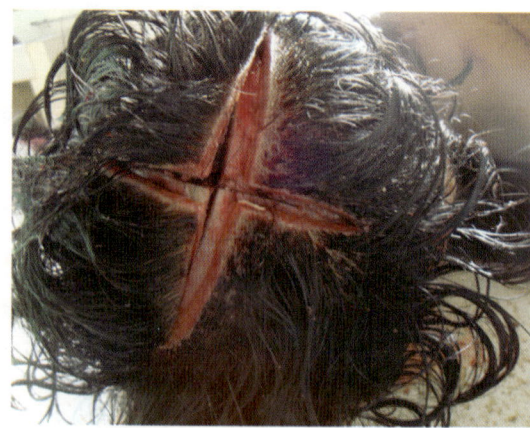

Fig. 3.13: Gaping incised wound

Fig. 3.14: Criss-cross gaping incised wound

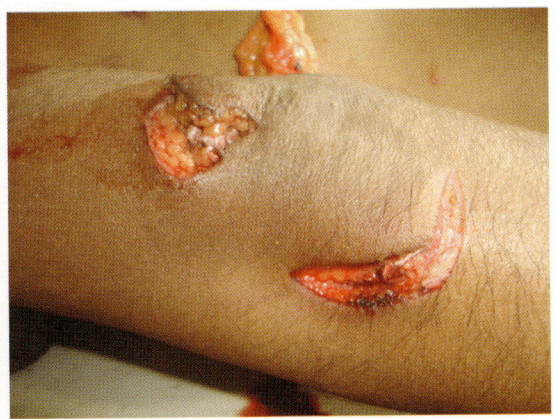

Fig. 3.15: Bevelled incised wound

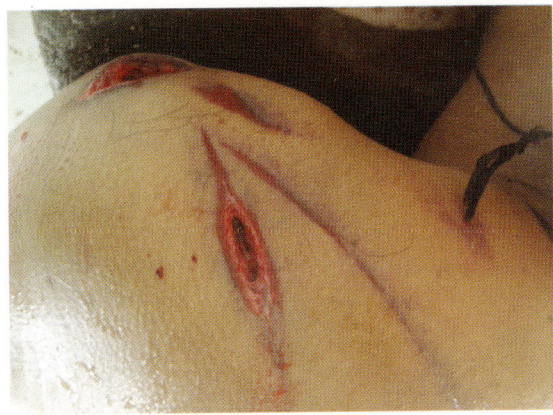

Fig. 3.16: Incised wound with tailing

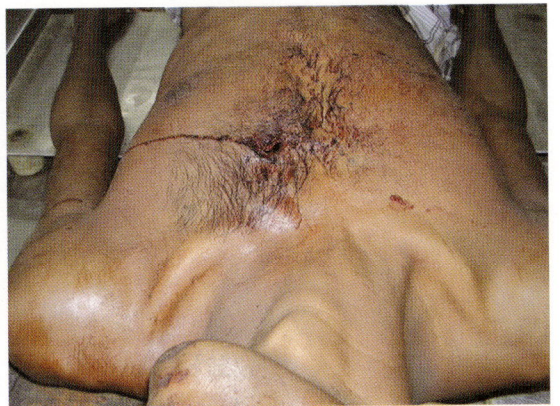

Fig. 3.17: Stab wound

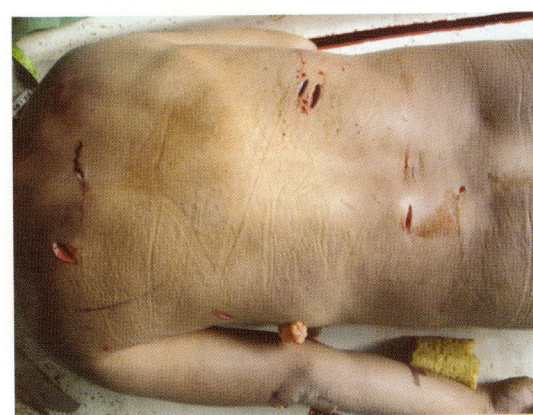

Fig. 3.18: Multiple stab wound

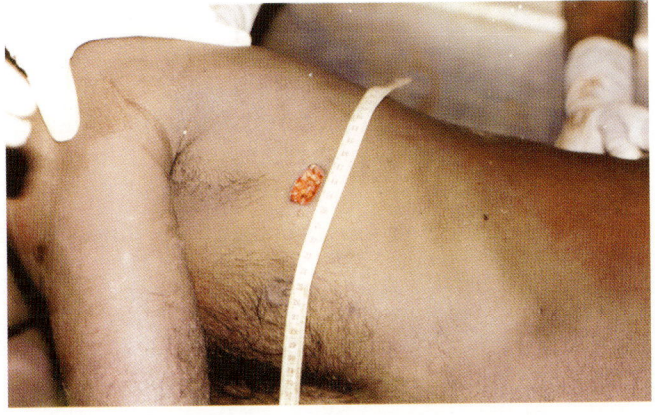

Fig. 3.19: Stab wound chest

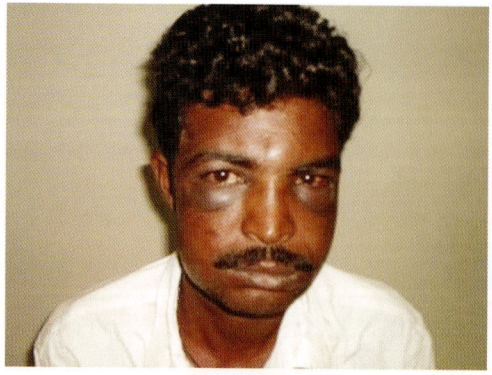

Fig. 3.20: Black eye

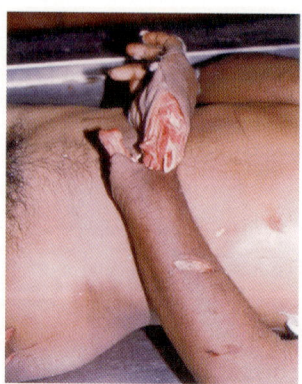

Fig. 3.21: Defence wound

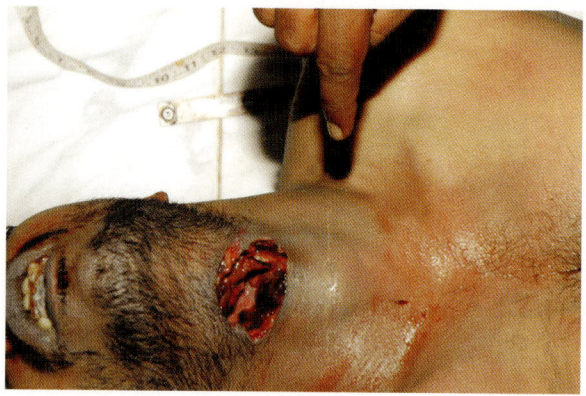

Fig. 3.22: Suicidal cut throat

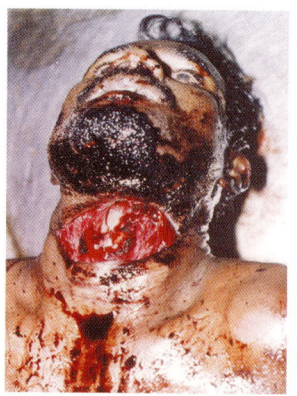

Fig. 3.23: Homicidal cut throat

EVALUATORY QUESTIONS

1. **Define a wound.**

   Legal definition: A wound is defined under Section 44 of IPC as any harm illegally caused to a person's body, mind, property or reputation.

   Medical definition: Any damage or discontinuity of any of the body tissues caused by application of force either deliberately or accidentally.

2. **Define hurt.**

   According to Section 319 IPC whoever causes bodily pain, illness or infirmity to any person is said to cause hurt.

3. **Define Grievous hurt.**

   According to Section 320 IPC, following kinds of hurt ONLY are designated as *grievous*:
   1. Emasculation (causing loss of libido)
   2. Permanent privation of the sight of either eye (loss of sight)
   3. Permanent privation of the hearing of either ear (loss of hearing)

4. Privation of any member or joint (severing a digit or limb)
5. Destruction or permanent impairing of the powers of any member or joint (incapacitation without severing)
6. Permanent disfiguration of the head or face (causing ugliness)
7. Fracture or dislocation of a bone or tooth (partial or complete fracture)
8. Any hurt which endangers life or which causes the injured to be in severe bodily pain or unable to follow his ordinary pursuits during the space of twenty days.

4. Define a simple wound.

Though it is not defined specifically in the IPC, a wound which is neither extensive nor grievous and heals readily without leaving a permanent scar or deformity or causing any functional impairment.

5. What is the etiological classification of wounds?

According to the source of energy, wounds are classified as *physical or mechanical injuries, chemical injuries, thermal injuries* and miscellaneous such as injuries due to electricity, explosion, lightening and radiation.

6. How are the mechanical injuries classified morphologically?

Mechanical injuries are classified broadly into two categories as *blunt force injuries* and *sharp force injuries*. Blunt force injuries are abrasions, contusions, lacerations, fracture of bones and crush injury. Sharp force injuries are incised wounds and punctured wounds which may be penetrating or perforating and also chop wounds, amputation and decapitation.

7. What is an abrasion?

Abrasion is a type of mechanical injury involving the epidermis alone caused by friction against any rough surface or object.

8. What is a contusion?

Contusion is a type of blunt force injury which is seen as discolouration of the skin over extravasated blood into tissue space due to capillovenous rupture.

9. What is a laceration?

Laceration is a type of blunt force injury resulting in forceful tear of skin and underlying tissues which are crushed between two hard objects, one is the weapon and another is the underlying bone.

10. How are the wounds classified clinically?

Clinically the wounds are classified as simple, grievous and dangerous in living persons.

11. How are the wounds classified medicolegally?

Wounds are classified medicolegally as suicidal, homicidal, accidental, fictitious or fabricated and defence wounds.

12. What are the legal responsibilities of the doctor in handling a seriously injured patient?

1. The doctor immediately informs the police officer particularly in assault cases.
2. If the wounds are very severe and life threatening, he arranges for recording the dying declaration by a Magistrate.

3. Before dying declaration is recorded he should certify the mental fitness of the injured.

4. If there is a delay in the arrival of the magistrate or if death is imminent, the doctor himself should record the declaration in the presence of two uninterested witnesses.

5. If the victim died, death should be intimated to the police, and death certificate must not be issued and body should be handed over to the police for autopsy.

13. What is a self-inflicted wound?

A self-inflicted wound is one which is caused by a person on himself.

The self-inflicted wound is categorized as suicidal, parasuicidal, psychotic and fictitious/ fabricated.

Suicidal wounds are throat cut injuries, wrist cutting or cuts over the groin or self-stab (Harakiri) wounds. These wounds are inflicted with an intention of killing oneself by causing injuries over vital areas.

Parasuicidal injuries are also self-inflicted wounds caused only to earn sympathy or to evade responsibility and are not usually life threatening.

Psychotic injuries are injuries which are inflicted by a person who has a psychotic disorder and are mostly mutilating in nature.

For example: Psychotic excoriations, delusion of parasitosis.

Lesch-Nyhan syndrome: Destructive lip/cheek biting due to familial disorder of uric acid metabolism.

Onychophagia: Nail biting

Bruxism: Grinding of teeth

Trichotillomania: Pulling of body hair

Thermophilia: Abnormal exposure of body parts to open fire or radiant heat

Fabricated or fictitious injuries: Injuries which are mostly self-inflicted or occasionally inflicted with the help of another person with a strong ulterior motive. The following are the usual motives for causing fabricated wounds.

1. To bring a false charge of assault against another person.

2. To escape a condition of stressful work, e.g. a soldier to avoid war duty

3. To be hospitalized, by a prisoner in order to escape being in prison.

4. To exaggerate or exacerbate the original lesion or injury, by industrial workers, to get more compensation under Workmen's Compensation Act (Benign self-mutilation or goldbricking)

5. To obliterate the personal identity in criminal cases by over tattooing or erasing the tattoo with caustics, destruction of fingerprint patterns by flame burns or chemical burns.

6. To support a false charge of sexual assault by a woman against an innocent male.

7. To support a concocted version of defence by police in cases of encounter deaths.

8. To escape suspicion or detection of deceitful act by connivance of criminals with security guards/police.

9. To mimic or simulate disease by employees so as to enjoy double benefits of long leave with salary (disability benefits).

For example, injecting air into subcutaneous tissue to mimic emphysema

Injecting milk subcutaneously to mimic disease of adipose tissue (factitial Weber-Christian syndrome).

14. What is an incised wound?

Incised wound is a type of sharp force injury resulting in clear division of skin and underlying soft tissues when the sharp edge of the weapon is drawn across the body surface.

15. Which type of laceration simulates an incised wound?

Split laceration is frequently mistaken as incised wound as there is no sufficient subcutaneous fat and soft tissue underneath the stretched skin which are typically seen over the scalp, chin, shin, etc.

16. What are the differences between an incised wound and lacerated wound?

S. No	Features	Lacerated wound	Incised wound
1	Type of force	Blunt force	Sharp force
2	Mechanism	Crushing of tissues	Clear division
3	Shape	Irregular	Usually spindle
4	Wound margin	Ragged	Smooth
5	Blood vessels	Crushed	Severed
6	Floor of the wound	Bridging tissues	No strands of tissues
7	Bleeding	Moderate	Profuse
8	Tissue damage	More (undermining)	Less (linear)
9	Hair bulb	Crushed	Severed
10	Healing	By secondary intention	Primary intention
11	Scar	Irregular	Linear

17. What are the differences between an incised wound and a stab wound?

S. No	Features	Incised wound	Stab wound
1	Wound mechanism	Linear division of skin with soft tissues by sharp edge	Forceful thrusting into the body tissues by sharp tip
2	Shape	Spindle or elliptical	Oval
3	Length	More than other dimension	Less than other dimension
4	Depth	Less than the length	More than the length
5	Gaping	Usual	Occasional
6	Manner	Usually self inflicted and fabricated, occasionally homicidal along with stabs	Usually homicidal, occasionally suicidal

18. What are the differences between suicidal and homicidal wounds?

S. No	Features	Suicidal	Homicidal
1.	Type of injury	Mostly incised or stab wounds rarely contusion or laceration	All types of wounds usually stab and chop wounds
2.	Site of injury	Only over accessible and vital areas such as neck, left chest and abdomen, sometimes over the great vessels in the wrist or groin	Anywhere on the body usually head, neck, chest and abdomen
3.	Number	Usually few	Usually multiple
4.	Direction	Always oblique from left to right or right to left depending upon right or left handedness. Downwards in the upper part of the body. Transverse in the abdomen. Upwards over the lower limbs	No specificity in directions.
5.	Secondary injuries	No other injuries	Associated injuries always present
6.	Hesitation injuries	Hesitation injuries always present	No hesitation or trial or tentative injuries
7.	Tailing/taper	Present if there is an incised wound	Occasionally present
8.	Beveling	Absent	Present
9.	Arrangement	Grouping of injuries at one site and superimposition of injuries noted	No such arrangement
10.	Defense injuries	No defence wounds	Defence wound may be present
11.	Signs of struggle	No signs of struggle	Struggle marks usually present
12.	Clothes	Clothes are not usually involved	Clothes overlying the injuries are usually damaged
13.	Circumstances	Secluded place	No preference
14.	Motive	Deep depression or dejection due to various causes	Usually enemity, revenge, etc.
15.	Weapon preferred	Sharp-edged light cutting weapon	Sharp-edged or moderately heavy cutting weapons or blunt weapons such as wooden log, crow bar or huge stone.
16.	Weapon in the scene	Always present, sometimes in tight grip (cadaveric spasm)	Weapon is not found, but rarely placed in hand to mimic cadaveric spasm
17.	Suicidal note	May be present	Never, may be planted to mislead.
18.	Foreign body	Absent	Foreign articles may be present at the scene. Foreign hair or shirt button may be present in the hand of the victim in a state of cadaveric spasm.

19. **Define a defence wound.**

    A wound sustained by a victim of assault by the instinctive act of retaliation by holding on to a weapon or to ward off an attack or by covering the vital part such as head, face, etc. to protect oneself from an assault. Types of defence wound depend on the nature of the weapon used.

    In case of blunt weapon such as wooden log, crow bar, iron pipe, brick or stone, injuries like abrasions, contusions, lacerations, nail break, avulsion or fracture of bones can occur.

    Example of patterned fracture in defense of being attacked with blunt weapons

    Bennett's intra-articular fracture of the first metacarpal bone.

    Night stick fracture of ulna at its end, by the downward moment of a club or stick.

    In case of sharp weapon such as knife, sickle, sword or axe being used, depending upon the act of self protection, the nature of the weapon and direction of assault, the type of injury results.

    For example, if the victim attempted to grasp the weapon, a linear deep cut over the palm in the case of single-edged knife and two parallel cuts involving the palm and flexures of the fingers are seen in case of double-edged knife.

    In an attempt to grasp a wielding sickle, cut injuries over the palm with complete or partial severance of the fingers can occur. When there is an attempt to ward off the attack by raising the hands, gaping incised wounds may be seen over the wrist or inner aspect of forearm with cut fracture of bones.

20. **What do you mean by dangerous weapon?**

    According to Section 324 IPC: Any instrument used for cutting, stabbing, shooting or any other instrument used as a weapon of offense is likely to cause death or by means of fire or any heated substance or by means of any poison or any corrosive substance or by means of any explosive substance or by means of any substance which is deleterious to the human body to inhale or ingest or to receive into the blood or by means of any animal shall be punished with imprisonment up to 3 years or with fine or with both.

21. **What do you mean by concealed puncture wounds?**

    Punctured wounds inflicted over hidden parts of the body in order to avoid suspicion or easy detection. The sites are fontanalle in infants, nape of neck in adults, nasal orifice, inner canthi of the eyes, urethral, anal or vaginal orifice, groin and axilla.

22. **What do you mean by *hidden contusion*?**

    Contusion of scalp tissue is not visible externally since it is hidden under the tuft of hair.

23. **What are the complications of injuries?**

    The immediate complications are shock, haemorrhage, air embolism. Intermediate complications are infection, sepsis, gangrene. Remote complications are scars with keloidal tendency, disability due to contracture or physical deformity, post-traumatic psychological disturbances.

LAWS RELATED TO PHYSICAL ASSAULT

Section 321 IPC: Voluntarily causing hurt

Section 322 IPC: Voluntarily causing grievous hurt

Section 323 IPC: **Punishment for causing hurt:** As per this Section, a person who has caused hurt voluntarily can be punished by a second class magistrate court by awarding up to 1 year imprisonment or fine of Rs. 1000 or both.

Section 324 IPC: Describes the dangerous weapons such as weapons of cutting, chopping, shooting or any instrument which is used as a weapon of offence or by means of explosives, fire, poisons, and animals or by means of any substance which is deleterious to human body. Anybody who voluntarily cause hurt on the person with such dangerous weapon can be punished by a first class magistrate up to 3 years imprisonment or with fine or with both.

Section 325 IPC: **Punishment for voluntarily causing grievous hurt:** Whoever causes grievous hurt voluntarily can be punished up to 7 years imprisonment by Chief Judicial Magistrate (CJM)/CMM.

Section 326 IPC: Punishment for causing grievous hurt with dangerous weapon, whoever voluntarily causes grievous hurt with dangerous weapon is punishable up to 10 years imprisonment by an Assistant Session Court.

Section 327 IPC: Voluntarily causing hurt to extort property or to constrain to an illegal act which is punishable up to 10 years.

Section 328 IPC: Causing hurt by means of poison, etc. with intent to commit an offence is punishable up to 10 years.

Section 351 IPC: **Assault:** Whoever makes any gesture or any preparation with an intention to cause apprehension of the person and believes that he is about to be attacked.

Section 352 IPC: Punishment for assault or criminal force other than on grave provocation can be imprisoned up to 3 months or 500 rupees or with both.

Section 353 IPC: Assault or criminal force to deter public servant from discharge of his duty is punishable up to 2 years imprisonment.

Section 354 IPC: Assault or criminal force to woman with intent to outrage her modesty is punishable up to 2 years or fine or with both.

Section 355 IPC: Assault or criminal force with intent to dishonor a person otherwise than on grave provocation is punishable up to 2 years.

Section 356 IPC: Assault or criminal force in attempt to commit theft of property carried by a person is punishable up to 2 years.

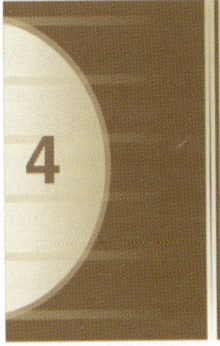

4   **Drunkenness Examination**

INTRODUCTION

Alcohol still holds the lead as the most common drug of abuse and it has been used for medicinal, religious and social purposes often inviting legal problems also. Alcohol is the product of fermentation of starch in the presence of yeast. It is characterised by a functional hydroxyl group (OH) attached to two carbon atoms (Fig. 4.1).

Ethyl alcohol or ethanol (C_2H_5OH) is meant for human consumption, the concentration of which varies in different types of alcoholic beverages. Ethanol is a colourless, volatile inflammable liquid emitting a strong fruity odour with a sweetish burning taste. The smell of alcohol is due to impurities (congeners) as higher alcohols like amyl and butyl alcohol, acetone and esters which are simultaneously produced during fermentation process.

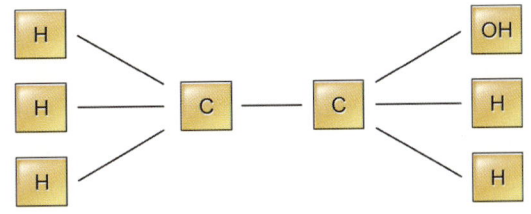

Fig. 4.1: Functional hydroxyl group attached to two carbon atoms

The purpose of distillation is only to increase the concentration of alcohol. The concentration of alcohol is being expressed in percentage by volume and according to this alcohol is classified as follows:

1. Absolute alcohol (99%)
2. Methylated alcohol (methanol) — (90% ethyl alcohol +10% methyl alcohol)
3. Rectified spirit (95% ethanol)
4. Surgical spirit (methylated spirit mixed with small amount of castor oil and methyl salicylate (winter green))
5. Proof spirit (mixture of alcohol and water in which the alcohol is 49.28% by weight or 57.10 by volume)
6. Fermented spirit (2 –10% ethanol)
7. Distilled spirit (40 – 50 % ethanol)

According to the percentage of alcohol, the beverages are broadly classified as:

1. Soft drink   Alcohol concentration 2 to 8 %
2. Moderate drink   Alcohol concentration 10 to 20%
3. Hard drink   Alcohol concentration 40 to 50 %

Absorption, Distribution and Elimination of Alcohol

Alcohol that is usually ingested is absorbed by simple diffusion from the mucosa of the stomach (20 – 25%) and from the upper part of small intestines (75–80%) mostly. The rate of absorption is influenced mainly by food contents in the stomach, gastric motility and pyloric function. Normally if alcohol is taken on an empty stomach it gets absorbed rapidly and reaches the peak level concentration within 30–45 minutes.

The rate of absorption is influenced by:

1. **Concentration that is consumed**: Generally, greater the concentration, faster it enters the bloodstream. (On the rocks is better than not on the rocks.)
2. **Nature of the mixing fluid**: Carbonated drink like soda promotes quick absorption than with plain water.
3. **State of the stomach**: Absorption is delayed by presence of food and quick absorption occurs in empty stomach.
4. **Condition of stomach**: Gastrectomy markedly accelerates the absorption as well as in chronic gastritis.
5. **Habit and tolerance**: Absorption occurs quickly in chronic drinkers than others.
6. **Emotional state**: Increases absorption by enhanced gastric emptying.
7. **Age**: Absorption occurs more quickly in older than young individuals.
8. **Sex**: Females get drunk faster than male.
9. **Drugs**: Atropine and benzedrine delays the absorption by reduced gastric motility.
10. **Rate of drinking**: Consumption of large quantity in short duration will delay the rate of absorption because of pylorospasm and vomiting.

The absorbed alcohol is carried to the liver by portal venous system where 90% of alcohol gets metabolised by the enzyme alcohol dehydrogenase into acetaldehyde and is catalysed by nicotinamide adenine dinucleotide (NAD). The resulting acetaldehyde is further oxidised by the enzyme aldehyde dehydrogenase into water and CO_2 with liberation of a little energy. The remaining 10% of unoxidised alcohol is transported by systemic circulation to all parts of the body. The concentration of alcohol occurs more in organs containing greater amount of water, especially the brain. Finally alcohol is excreted mainly through kidneys, alveoli and sweat and salivary glands to a lesser extent.

The rate of metabolism in the liver is estimated around (10–15 mg/hour/100 ml) and it normally requires 12 hours for a person to become sober after consumption of alcohol.

Effects of Alcohol

Alcohol is a depressant causing an irregular descending depression of the nervous system. First the reticular activating system is depressed, hence control of the higher centre over the lower centres is lost and leads to *release phenomena*. This release phenomena is responsible for the false sense of well being, increase in sociability, overconfidence, not cautious, emotionally unstable with enhanced aggression and often quarrelsome.

Next cortical depression occurs with motor and then the sensory cortex resulting in sensory and motor disturbances.

Then in descending order the cerebellum and spinal cord sparing the midbrain are affected and finally the pons with excessive consumption. When the cerebellum is affected, there is a disturbance in the gait and when the spinal cord is affected, disturbances in deep reflexes and muscular incoordination result.

Finally the midbrain is depressed resulting in vomiting, miosis, disturbance of consciousness, hypothermia, labouring breath, incontinence of urine and motion and if not treated at this stage death ensues either due to respiratory failure or circulatory failure or due to depression of cardiorespiratory centre in the midbrain or sometimes asphyxia due to falling back of tongue or aspiration of gastric contents. People recovering from deadly effects experience temporary aversion to alcohol due to disturbing residual effects (hangover), but unfortunately they again get back to drinking.

In the gastrointestinal tract low concentration of alcohol increases the appetite, moderate concentration promotes absorption and intoxication and high concentration causes gastric erosion and pylorospasm.

Alcohol is a vasodilator in moderate quantity but when consumed in excessive amounts, it causes peripheral circulatory collapse. Body becomes warm initially yet hypothermia is the terminal effect of excessive consumption.

Tolerance is an important ingredient for addiction since there is a compulsive increase in quantity of consumption to obtain the required effect on regular and repeated indulgence.

Psychological and social adaptability is directly affected by increasing concentration of alcohol in the blood and brain. According to the deviation of behavioural pattern and organic disturbances, the effects of alcohol are explained in three stages:

1. Stage of excitation
2. Stage of intoxication or in-coordination
3. Stage of coma

In modern days with changing culture alcohol has been accepted as a social antidote suitable for both joyful and sorrowful occasions. The following behavioural disorders with graded blood alcohol concentration (BAC) are fractioned in seven stages for practical purposes.

1. Stage of sobriety
2. Stage of euphoria
3. Stage of excitation
4. Stage of confusion
5. Stage of stupor
6. Stage of coma
7. Stage of death

"Drunkenness Does not Create Vices But Brings them to the Fore"—Seneca

Frequently doctors especially CMOs are requested by the police to examine an individual who has by his disorderly behaviour created public nuisance or by rash driving endangered public safety, or assaulted or attempted to murder or rape. In all these cases it is the duty of every medical officer not only to ascertain the degree of intoxication but also to prevent death when the individual is grossly intoxicated.

The degree of intoxication can be assessed by clinical examination with supportive laboratory investigations. The behaviour of a drunken person is determined by the blood alcohol concentration; invariably BAC always correlates with clinical findings. According to the blood alcohol concentration (which is normally expressed in mg/litre of blood), the clinical findings can be described in seven stages (Table 4.1).

A person is said to be drunk when he is so much under the influence of alcohol as to have lost control of faculties to such an extent as to render him unable to execute safely the occupation in which he is engaged at the material time.   — by Spl. Committee of BMA in 1927

Definition of Drunkenness

Drunkenness is a clinical condition resulting from excessive consumption of alcohol to such an extent as to have lost control over his/her faculties which renders him/her unable to execute the job safely at the material time.

STAGES OF ALCOHOLIC INTOXICATION

Table 4.1: Seven stages of alcoholic intoxication

Sl.	BAC mg/100 ml	Stage	Affected site of CNS	Clinical findings	Behaviour
1.	Up to 50 mg	Sobriety	Nil	Smell of alcohol in breath, suffused eyes, facial flushing	Decent
2.	50–100 mg	Euphoria	Reticular activating system Paradoxical stimulation of lower centres by phenomena release	Sense of well being, increased self-confidence, lower caution. Decreased inhibitions. Dilated pupil but brisk to light reflex.	Delighted
3.	100–150 mg	Excitation	Frontal lobe and parietal lobe	Emotional instability, difficulty in skillful activities, impaired memory. Increase in reaction time, dilated pupils—diminished light reflex, nystagmus	Devilish
4.	150–200 mg	Confusion	Occipital lobe, temporal lobe, thalamus and hypothalamus, limbic area	Blurred vision (diplopia), disorientation, confusion, in-coordination of thought, act and speech, impaired judgement	Dazed
5.	200–300 mg	Stupor	Cerebellum and spinal cord	Marked muscular in-coordination, inability to stand or walk, staggering gait, diminished reflexes, hiccups	Dejected
6.	300–500 mg	Coma	Medullary centres	Unconsciousness, vomiting, respiratory difficulty (stertorous breathing) hypothermia, hypotension, pinpoint pupil, abolished reflexes	Dead drunk
7.	>500 mg	Death	Paralysis of respiratory centre	Death due to respiratory paralysis	Dead

Drunkenness per se is unquestionable or punishable but performing certain acts or violating the public tranquillity or the statutory law invites stringent action.

To certify a state of drunkenness, the doctor should have a thorough knowledge about the intoxicating effects of ethyl alcohol, which can be easily described in the seven stages of intoxication (Table 4.1).

Alcohol produces irregular descending depression and recovery takes place in reversal order.

Scheme of examination

1. Authorisation
2. Preliminary data
   Name: .... Age: .... Sex: ....
   Address: .... Occupation: ....
   Identification marks:
         1.
         2.
3. Precaution
       Informed consent:
       Date, time and place of examination:
       Brought by:
4. History
   Has he consumed alcohol? If yes, quality, quantity, mixing (diluted or not) relation to food. Is he a habitual drinker, if so, since how long and how frequently he drinks?
5. Medical history
   Is he suffering from diabetes, hypertension, epilepsy, had he undergone any abdominal surgery?
6. Rule out the conditions of apparent alcoholism
   - Head injury
   - Epilepsy
   - Diabetes ⟨ Hypo / Hyper ⟩ glycemia
   - Parkinsonism
   - Disseminated sclerosis
   - Drug intoxication
   - Uraemic coma, hepatic coma
   - Snake bite
7. General examination
   Pulse, BP, temperature, CVS, RS, ABD. Appearance: State of clothing, hair.
8. Specific examination
   Behaviour : Cooperative, evasive or abusive
   Speech   : Normal, slurred and incoherent
   Orientation: Time, space
   Memory   : Recent and remote

Eyes:
>   State of conjunctiva:
>   State of pupil:
>   Light and accommodation reflex:
>   Movements of eyeball (lateral nystagmus):
>   Visual acuity:

Mouth:
>   State of lips and tongue:
>   Salivation:

Breath:
>   Smell of alcohol
>   Muscular coordination:
>   Finger to fingers:
>   Finger to nose:
>   Reaction time:
>   Stance Romberg's sign:
>   Gait:

Reflexes:
>   Normal or depressed:

9. Laboratory investigations
>   Blood 10 ml blood in sodium fluoride
>   Urine 30 ml of urine (second sample) phenylmercuric nitrate

10. Opinion

On the basis of the above observations, I am of the opinion that
(a) The person has consumed alcohol and is under its influence
(b) The person has consumed alcohol but not under the influence
(c) The person has not consumed alcohol.

> Signature of Medical Officer
> Registration No...................

Date:

Place:

JUSTIFICATION

- No smell with normal findings: Not consumed
- Smell with normal findings clinically: Consumed but not under influence
- Smell with abnormal clinical findings: Consumed and under influence
- Positive laboratory report is supportive evidence.

EVALUATORY QUESTIONS

1. **What is drunkenness?**

Drunkenness is a clinical condition resulting from excessive consumption of alcohol to such an extent as to have lost control over his/her faculties which renders him/her unable to execute the job safely at the material time.

2. **What are the different types of alcohol?**
   Ethanol, methanol, isoprophyl alcohol, butyl alcohol and amyl alcohol.

3. **Which type of alcohol is meant for human consumption?**
   Ethyl alcohol is meant for human consumption.

4. **What are the different forms of ethyl alcohol?**
   According to the concentration, the ethyl alcohol is termed into
   1. Absolute alcohol (99%)
   2. Methylated alcohol (methanol—90% ethyl alcohol +10% methyl alcohol)
   3. Rectified spirit (95% ethanol)
   4. Surgical spirit (methelated spirit mixed with small amount of castor oil and methyl salicylate (winter green))
   5. Proof spirit (mixture of alcohol and water in which the alcohol is 49.28% by weight or 57.10 by volume)
   6. Fermented spirit (2–10% ethanol)
   7. Distilled spirit (40–50% ethanol)

5. **What are the different types of alcoholic beverages?**
   According to the percentage of ethyl alcohol, the alcoholic beverages are classified as
   (a) Fermented beverages: Toddy—2 to 4%
   Bear—2 to 8%
   Wine—10–15%
   Fortified wine—15–20%
   (b) Distilled spirit: Obtained by evaporation and condensation of fermented spirit in order to increase the concentration of alcohol.
   Arrack (country liquor), brandy, whisky, gin (40–45%), rum, vodka (45–50%)

6. **How the ingested alcohol absorbs into the system?**
   20% of the consumed alcohol absorbed from the stomach and 80% from the intestine.

7. **How long after the first dose of alcohol consumed reaches the blood?**
   Alcohol can be detected in the blood usually after 30–45 minutes depends upon several factors such as dilution, state of stomach, presence of food, etc.

8. **How the alcohol is metabolised in the body?**
   Alcohol is metabolised in the liver mainly by first into acetaldehyde by alcohol dehydrogenase enzyme, next the acetaldehyde into carbondioxide and water by aldehyde dehydrogenase enzyme and the two metabolic process is catalysed by nicotinamide adenine dinucleotide.

9. **What is the mechanism of action of alcohol in the body?**
   Alcohol has got a depressive effect over the central nervous system in irregular descending fashion.

10. **What is the pharmacological effect of alcoholic consumption?**
    In less dosage it increases the appetite, elevates the mood, dilates the pupil (pseudo excitement—euphoria).

11. What are the toxicological effects?

In large dosage it causes gastric erosion, excitation, aggression, confusion, muscular inco-ordination, gait disturbance, hypothermia, stupor, constricted pupil, coma and death due to failure of cardiorespiratory centres in the medulla.

12. What do you mean by apparent alcoholism?

Exhibiting certain signs of alcoholism without consumption of alcohol is known as apparent alcoholism.

13. What are the conditions which mimicks alcoholism?

The following are the conditions which mimicks alcoholism commonly.

1. Epilepsy
2. Head injury
3. Intoxication with narcotics
4. Meningitis
5. Diabetes mellitus
6. Parkinsonism
7. Multiple sclerosis

14. What is nystagmus?

Nystagmus is the term applied to a disturbance of ocular movements characterised by involuntary and rhythmical oscillation of the eyeballs.

15. How to demonstrate the nystagmus?

Nystagmus can be demonstrated by asking the patient to sit at 1½ feet away from you. Ask him to look at your left eye with his right eye while his left eye is covered with his left hand and keep your hand midway between you and him. Ask him to look at your hand and follow your hand without moving his head in all the directions, i.e. horizontal (right to left) and vertical (up and down). By making this, only the eyes alone is moving and the movement of the eyeball is carried out by six extraocular muscles. The lateral rectus is supplied by 6th cranial nerve and superior oblique is supplied by 4th cranial nerve and other four muscles are supplied by 3rd cranial nerve. Incoordination of movement of eyeball occurs due to alcoholic intoxication resulting in oscillatory movement of the eyeball in a particular direction especially in lateral direction which is a sign of alcohol intoxication.

16. What are the points to be observed in the examination of eyes?

1. Corneal reflex
2. State of conjunctiva
3. Pupillary size on both eyes
4. Light reflex and accommodation reflex on both eyes
5. Nystagmus
6. McEwan sign

17. What is McEwan sign?

In acute alcoholic intoxication initially the pupil is dilated but when the person becomes comatose pupil becomes constricted. When skin is pinched over the neck or slapped over the cheek this constricted pupil gets dilated and again constricted when the stimulus is withdrawn. This is carried by cervical sympathetic nerve. This sign is useful to differentiate alcoholic coma from other causes of coma.

18. **What is Romberg sign?**

Romberg sign is a test for cerebellar function. When alcohol is consumed in excess, it depresses the cerebellar functions and takes away the positional sense, hence the person is unable to maintain erect posture with close feet and closed eyes.

19. **How to examine Romberg sign?**

Ask the person to stand erect with close feet and adducted hands with eyes open for sometime, then ask him to close his eyes and observe him whether he is steady or sway to one or other side or front or back (positive Romberg sign).

20. **What is hangover syndrome?**

Physical distress followed by excessive consumption of alcohol characterised by headache, nausea, vomiting and fatigue.

21. **What is alcoholic blackout?**

Transient anterograde amnesia (alcoholic blackout) in which the person forgets all or part of what happened during excessive consumption.

22. **What is micturition syncope?**

Loss of consciousness during the act of micturition after heavily drunk due to orthosatic hypotension caused by pooling of blood in the dilated peripheral veins after raises up suddenly from the bed.

23. **What is tolerance?**

Tolerance is the cellular adaptation to steadily increasing intake of intoxicating agents including alcohol.

24. **What is dipsomania?**

Irresistible desire to drink alcohol repeatedly.

25. **What is a delirium tremens?**

A state of psycho-somatic disorders with disturbed consciousness associated with mental confusion, agitation, emotional instability, insomnia, tachycardia, hypertension, tremors associated with horrifying hallucinations and delirium followed by sudden withdrawal of alcohol.

26. **Which section of IPC empowered to detain a person who creates nuisance in the public under the influence of alcohol?**

Section 510 IPC empowers to detain an individual creating public nuisance under the influence of alcohol who can be imprisoned for 24 hours or fine of Rs 10 or with both.

27. **Which section of IPC deals with criminal responsibility of an inebriated person who has committed an offence?**

IPC Section 85 deals with criminal responsibility of involuntary alcoholism as nothing is an offence which is done by a person who at the time of doing it is by reason of intoxication, incapable of knowing the nature of the act or that he is doing what is either wrong or contrary to law, provided that the thing which intoxicated him was administered to him without his knowledge or against his will. IPC Section 86 deals with voluntary alcoholism where a person who does an act in a state of intoxication shall be liable for his act if he has done with intention and knowledge as he would have had if he had not been intoxicated.

28. **What is a holiday heart?**

Transient paroxysmal tachycardia occurs after taking alcohol in certain individual who have no other evidence of heart disease.

29. **What is Widmark's formula?**

Widmark's formula is useful to estimate the total amount of alcohol consumed from blood alcohol concentration. It is a back calculation formula as

a = pcr, where

a—total amount of alcohol in gm percentage

p—weight of the individual in kilograms

c—blood alcohol concentration in mgms percentage

r—constant factor 0.6 for men and 0.5 for women

30. **Which section of Indian Motor Vehicle Act prescribes punishment for drunken drive?**

Section 185 of Indian Motor Vehicle Act prescribes a fine up to Rs 2000 for drunken drive.

31. **What are the congeners?**

Congeners are impurities which are the by-products of fermentation; they are traces of methanol, amyl and butyl alcohol, aldehydes and esters. These congeners are responsible for imparting the characteristic smell of alcohol, which may persist even after complete elimination of alcohol from the body.

32. **What are the important responsibilities of examining doctor before issuing opinion on the state of an intoxicated person?**

- Obtain consent
- Examine head to toe to assess his mental, physical and behavioural pattern which is markedly affected by ethanol.
- Corroborate the clinical features to assess whether the person is merely consumed alcohol or under its influence.
- Collection of blood and urine should be done after explaining the purpose and also the outcome under consent. However, the positive results are the proof of consumption.
- Although smell of alcohol in breath and suffusion of eyes are proof of consumption but not sufficient to declare as under the influence of alcohol.

EXERCISE

Govindan, 35 years old, male, S/O Sundaran residing at 11, Gandhi St., Guduvanchery, was brought at 8 PM on 20.06.07 by head constable no. 303, Muthiah of Guduvanchery Police Station with a police memo No. 48/2007 dated 20.06.07 issued by the Subinspector of Police Guduvanchery Police Station with alleged history of disorderly behaviour and causing annoyance to the public in bus stand.

The following are the findings of clinical examination.

1. Uncooperative and abusive behaviour.
2. Congested eyes, dilated pupil sluggishly reacting to light, lateral nystagmus.
3. Memory for recent and remote events impaired.
4. Speech slurred.
5. Staggering gait.
6. Positive Romberg's sign.
7. Breath strong odour of alcohol.

Identification Marks

1. A black mole on top of right shoulder
2. A black mole on front of right side chest

How will you proceed with examination and issue a certificate regarding his degree of drunkenness?

Register No. ....

Department of Forensic Medicine
Drunkenness—Examination Proforma

Requisition from the Judicial Magistrate of/Inspector of ....
vide letter/crime no. .... dated.....................

1. Name of the individual   :
2. Sex   :
3. Residential address   :
4. Occupation   :
5. Age   :
6. Persons accompanying or brought by :
7. Time, date and place of examination :
8. Consent of the individual for examination :
9. Marks of identification
    1.
    2.
10. History
    Present:
    Past:
    Medical:
11. General examination
    Pulse: /mt   B.P: /   mm of Hg
    C.V.S:
    R.S:
    Abd.
    C.N.S:
12. Appearance and behaviour   Normal/tidy/co-operative/abusive/evasive
13. Higher functions   :   Speech: Orientation:
                                          Memory:
14. Examination of eyes   :
        Conjunctivae   :
        Pupil   :   Size: Light reflex:
                                          Accommodation reflex:
        Visual field (ocular movement) :
15. Examination of mouth   :   State of tongue and lips
16. Breath   :
17. Reflexes   :
18. Muscular co-ordination   :
19. Gait   :
20. Investigations   :
21. Opinion   :

Place: Signature
Date:

Register No. ....

Department of Forensic Medicine

Drunkenness Certificate

I Dr .... have examined a person of a male/female calling himself/herself .... age stated .... years an inhabitant of .... bearing the following identification marks.

        1.

        2.

on .... at .... am/pm.

Based on the clinical findings of his/her examination, I am of the opinion that

  (a) He/she has consumed alcohol and under its influence.

  (b) He/she has consumed alcohol but not under its influence.

  (c) He/she has not consumed alcohol.

Station: Signature

Date:

Justification in support of the opinion given

1.

2.

3.

4.

5.

5   Sexual Offence—Examination

INTRODUCTION

Incomplete knowledge about the anatomical and physiological changes during sexual union of male and female is the commonest reason for a misleading conclusion regarding medico-legal opinion in cases of sexual assault, resulting in miscarriage of justice. Like any other medicolegal examination involving a living individual, examination of victim/assailant of sexual assault is also the same. It needs an intimate examination and evaluation of anogenital region to assess the normal development and also to ascertain the evidence of union of genital organs of the involved parties. A written informed consent is most important to avoid allegation of tort or criminal force upon the doctor at a later date. Apart from this legal precaution a doctor must realize that his/her opinion is a corroborative evidence to conform or to confront the victim's claim. As the sexual offences never used to have ocular witnesses a meticulous medical opinion alone can help the law courts to penalize the culprit as well as set free the innocent. Hence a sound knowledge in anatomy of genital organs and applied aspect of each and every part of the genital and accessory organ system is essential to appreciate the truthfulness of the victim's complaint against accused/suspected person. Ignorance/ inexperience and lack of interest among the doctors lead to denial of justice to a poor victim or wrongful conviction of an innocent suspect. To avoid miscarriage of justice one should refresh the genital anatomy and its application to solve the sensational legal problem.

FEMALE GENITAL ANATOMY

Vulva, otherwise known as pudendum, is the most secret and protected part of female extending between mons pubis in front and anus behind and genitocrural folds on either side.

Medicolegal Importance of Vulva

Vulva is supposed to be an erogenous zone with enriched blood and nerve supply. Any physical (digital or instrumental), oral or penile intervention leaves some signs in the form of abrasions or contusions and bite mark commonly and laceration rarely. Other than these, physical evidences such as fibre, hair and body fluids such as blood, saliva and semen may also present over this region. Hence it is very important to observe and evaluate this region before proceeding further in a case of sexual assault case.

Furthermore, the pubic hair which is abundant over the mons pubis grown in a triangular fashion with the base over the mons downwards over the labium majora. Growth of pubic hair in female usually occurs between 12 and 14 years, a few of which may fall daily as like hair on other parts of the body. The pubic hair must be combed to find out lose hair which may belong to the accused, a proof of union. Sometimes fiber or fabric, gravel or gross dust may also be adherent to the pubic hair. Apart from the above blood, saliva or seminal fluid may be soaked into the pubic hair by which the pubic hair becomes adherent with each other as tuft (matted). This matted hair must be preserved for detection of source and its biological identity. Control for comparison must be collected from the victim by plucking the pubic and scalp hair and blood and saliva over filter paper or dried clean cotton ball.

Vestibule

It is an oval-shaped cleft in middle of the vulva also known as pudendal cleft extending from the clitoris in front to the fourchette at the rear and laterally bounded by folds of (connective tissue and skin) labium minora and majora on either side. The vestibule is harbouring one urethral opening in front and vaginal opening behind. These important urogenital openings are guarded by thick skin fold outside (labium majora) and soft connective tissue fold (labium minora) inside. Apart from the urethral and vaginal openings, duct of Bartholin glands and para urethral glands (Skene's duct) also opens into the vestibule. The vestibule is wet due to mucus secretion and warm because of abundant blood supply. This important area is normally covered by its outer lip, the labium majora on either side which are firmly in contact at the midline and non-separable even on extreme abduction of thighs usually in virgin girls and requires digital separation for penile penetration at the time of first coitus. As the vestibule is richly supplied with venous plexus even a trivial pressure either with digit or penis can lead to congestion/hyperaemia.

MEDICOLEGAL EXAMINATION OF VICTIM OF SEXUAL ASSAULT: GENERAL EXAMINATION

Introduction

Sexual assault is a violent crime against woman and children of all ages. This is the only crime usually committed in the absence of third person; hence there is no eye (ocular) witness for this serious crime. But frequently complaints of sexual assault are brought to the limelight only after detection by the mother of the victim or other relatives. Sometimes, false charge of sexual assault are being brought with an ulterior motive of matrimonial or monetary gain. It is not uncommon that female children are portrayed as victims of sexual abuse in order to avenge for personal or professional rivalry. Hence, any woman approaching a police or a doctor or any other responsible citizen, with history of allegation of sexual assault should be immediately subjected to medical examination. The medical examination is mandatory to corroborate the allegation of sexual assault with the subjective signs and objective evidences of sexual union along with retrieval of trace evidence as proof of scientific evidence. Sexual union can be established easily by medical examination when it is performed as early as possible after the act, otherwise biological and physical trace evidences will gradually disappear as the time passes. A detailed history about the offence is mandatory which should comprise the day, time, location and individual or individuals involved and whether the act was consensual or nonconsensual. The details about the sexual intercourse such as position of act, with or without clothes, degree of intermission, emission, attainment of orgasm and reaction of the victim during the entire process and also postcoital activities should be recorded. In sexual history details of exposure to intercourse before and after the occurrence of present allegation must be elicited. Unless it has been elicited in detail, it is highly impossible to corroborate with the findings of general and genital examination.

Why the Victim of Sexual Assault should be Examined?

From medicolegal point of view when the rights and freedom of a woman is deprived and disregarded by a man either forcibly or deceitfully to have sexual intercourse it amounts to heinous felony. However, on many occasions this inviolable act is not being reported immediately and hence it becomes more difficult either to conclude or confront the allegation of sexual assault on a female by a male. Though severe punitive laws have been in force to prevent the sinful crime against womanhood of any age, lack of skill in examination and lassitude among the doctors while deposing in a court of law as an expert witness has contributed in miscarriage of justice. A meticulous medical examination alone can confirm or rule out the sexual union between a male and female, without which many fictitious allegation of sexual assault may invite punishment of innocent male. Hence doctors should not evade their legal obligation in carrying out a diligent evaluation, interpretation of examination findings scientifically with corroboration of analytical reports and circumstances. Only a systematic scientific examination can enable them to boldly face a judicial trial.

What are the Biological Evidences of Sexual Intercourse from the Victim?

1. Hair—body hair or pubic hair belonging to the accused: A careful inspection and combing of pubic hair may be helpful to retrieve hair of the accused. This may be lost by removing the panties or during wash or bath.
2. Whitish discharge per vagina: All whitish discharge per vagina need not necessarily be seminal fluid since leucorrhoea due to various causes may be frequently present. However, detection of spermatozoa in the vagina is a conclusive proof of sexual union. This cellular component of seminal fluid is quickly lost in several ways such as natural drain, urination, douching and bathing. The sperms ejaculated into the vagina have limited survival period due to acidic environment of the vaginal secretion (motile sperm can be detected up to 6 hours after the ejaculation, non-motile sperm up to 12 hours and disintegrated sperm up to 24 hours in the vaginal canal).

   The fluid part of seminal fluid is mainly formed by prostatic secretion and it can be detected up to 36 to 48 hours.

What are the Aims of Examination?

1. Evaluation of the incident
2. Examination to assess the general and genital injury and to alleviate the pain and suffering
3. Evidence collection to identify suspect
4. Prevention of sexually transmitted disease/pregnancy
5. Psychological support
6. Preparation of document for offering opinion.

What are the Important Requirements for Examination?

1. Authorization: Normally a requisition from a police officer not below the rank of sub-inspector or a magistrate can authorize the examination if it has already been reported, if not, the doctor must immediately examine and subsequently inform the police (according to 39 CrPC) when the victim reports to the doctor directly. The doctor should not refuse the examination for want of requisition, thereby causing loss of all the trace evidences in proving the sexual assault.

2. Confirm the identity of the individual to be examined by comparing the identification marks noted by the requesting authority.

3. Consent for examination: Though the consent of the victim is implied a written consent after discussing nature of physical examination is explained is to be obtained. If the victim is incompetent to give consent due to her age (below 12 years) or is mentally unsound, consent must be obtained from the parent or guardian. The examination should be conducted in a closed room with adjustable focus lamp, adequate instruments and ensure privacy without discomfort either to the victim or to the doctor.

4. Witness for examination: During the examination, especially when carried out by a male doctor presence of a disinterested female witness is always safe to avoid embarrassing allegations of tort or criminal intimidation. A female nurse is preferable and should be present throughout the examination and never allow victim's relative during the examination.

How to Proceed with Examination?

1. Personal data such as name, age, address, occupation and marital status are to be recorded.

2. Name and number of the police personnel who brought or the accompanied relatives of the victim should also be recorded.

3. Note down two identification marks which are consistent with the identification given in the requisition and if there is inconsistency, inform the police personnel to correct the same.

4. Consent: Written informed consent must be obtained.

5. Record physical status such as height, weight, chest and abdominal girth, hair growth and dental pattern.

6. History evaluation: Win the confidence of the victim by being sympathetic and have an empathic approach so as to elicit as much information as possible without embarrassment or concealment. The most important Ws are When, Where and Who. The time, day and date, place of occurrence and sexual assault by known or unknown person or persons should be recorded. Then the details such as indoor or outdoor, if indoor in whose house, any other person present there, did she accept or object, did she resist or raise hue or cry, and did he force or threatened her must be recorded. Was she in her full senses or under the influence of drinks or drugs? Was she completely clothed or not and the position of the victim during the act. Whether the penetration was vulval or vaginal? Did he ejaculate inside or outside vagina, did she attain orgasm, her behaviour following the act—whether she rose up immediately or not, whether she washed or wiped her genital? Whether she passed urine or taken bath? All these details should be elicited for corroborating with the findings and to retrieve the remnant of biological trace evidences in and around the genitalia.

Did she report immediately after the incident or detected by relatives and subsequently reported? If there is any delay in reporting, reason for the delay should also be sought. All these details should be recorded in verbatim and if there is any inconvincible point the same should be clarified. Apart from the history of the incident, the past history briefly covering the medical history (illness, injury and medication), menstrual history (age of menarche, frequency and regularity), sexual history (exposure prior and after the incident), marital and parital history, if married, must also be recorded.

General Examination

1. To assess the physical ability to offer resistance
2. To document the signs of struggle/violence
3. To correlate the alleged age
4. To retrieve the trace evidences

The physical ability of the victim can be assessed with physical development by measuring the height, weight, shoulder breadth, chest and abdominal girth and nutritional status by body built.

The important objective of general examination is to appreciate and to document the objective evidences of physical violence in the form of abrasion, contusion, laceration, fist and bite marks over the face, around mouth, neck, breast, arms, abdomen, thighs and pressure parts such as back of shoulders, elbow, buttocks, calves and heels. Lips, teeth, nails should be examined with special attention. Whenever there is an open injury, it should be entered into accident register and a wound certificate also must be issued.

The next important aspect of general examination is to correlate the stated age of the victim with physical, dental and sexual maturity indicators.

The physical measurements already recorded along with the dental pattern, developmental state of breast and external genital organs and hair growth should be documented. If there is no documentary proof for age or the alleged age is grossly discriminate with appearance, radiological assessment must also be done along with physical and dental examinations.

The next important aspect of general examination is to look for trace evidences found on the body which may connect to place of occurrence as well as the accused person involved. If such evidences are detected they should be retrieved, documented and preserved properly for further analysis.

The non-biological evidences may be dust, grass, gravel, sand, fibre, fabrics, etc. and biological trace evidences such as hair, saliva, blood, seminal fluid (fresh or dried) and nails scrapings (may contain epithelial debris or blood pigments of accused) must be collected using a tooth pick from each finger separately particularly when there is history of scratch over the face or body of the accused in an attempt to prevent his advancement.

If there is bite mark, differentiate whether it is love bite or chew bite by the size, site, shape and depth of teeth impressions with defect in the skin. All the above findings of bite marks are determined by mechanism of force either sucking force (love bite) or crushing force (true bite).

Take photography with measuring scale in right position. Collect saliva by using sterile cotton swab after which acrylic cast must be prepared without delay for comparison with the dental cast of alleged/suspected individual.

The extremities also must be looked for evidence of bonding (ligature mark) around wrist and ankle in case of gang rape. The victim must also be examined for evidence of drugs or drinks which may be given to her deceitfully by the accused.

The last but not the least is the examination of clothes. If the victim has not changed the clothes which she was wearing at the time of the incident it should be examined for signs such as tear, defect, loss of hook or button, trace evidences such as hair, stains of blood, semen and saliva over the undergarments, if such findings are detected that should be documented, preserved and forwarded to the forensic laboratory for further analysis. Finally the gait of the victim must be observed and recorded as there is a possibility of difficulty in walking due to forcible sexual intercourse usually in gang rape.

Genital Examination

After a thorough general examination, genital examination should be commenced in the examination room of the hospital/department observing proper precautions. Though the examination is similar to a gynecological examination, the manner and method is entirely different in case of sexual assault examination. Visual examination is more vital than the palpable examination observed from superficial to deep structures. The genital examination determines evidences of sexual assault with subjective structural damage and elements of trace evidences. The examination must be carried out in lithotomy position with a good source of light (focus light) and with proper instrumental facilities as magnifying lens with illumination facility, sterile gloves, speculum, sterile swabs, pipette, saline, glass slides, etc.

Dictum to be Remembered in Genital Examination

1. A lady MO should only examine the alleged rape victim. However, if on that particular day and time, a female MO is not available, a male MO should examine the victim in the presence of a female nurse/attendant.

2. Never touch the genitals without prior consent and proper privacy for visual examination.

3. The genital findings are influenced by the following factors

   (a) Age: Severity or degree of genital damage is directly proportional to the disparity in size of female to male genital organ. Thus a child victim sustains severe genital injury as compared to an adult female while an elderly victim will also sustain severe damage similar to child victim because of senile atrophic changes.

   (b) Frequency of sexual exposure: A woman accustomed to frequent sexual intercourse sustains less or no injury when compared to a virgin whose genitals show severe damage.

   (c) Time lapsed after last coitus: Due to healing process the injuries are likely to gradually disappear with the passage of time following the last act of coitus.

   (d) Retrieval of trace evidences also decreases with increase in time lapse after sexual intercourse

   (e) Hymenal tear alone, in the absence of local or general injuries, in a virgin is not a proof of rape.

(f) Intact hymen does not exclude rape since intercourse is possible by vulval penetration. The hymen stretches sufficiently to accommodate the erected penis without undergoing damage.

(g) Document all the findings of your examination including all negative findings.

Steps of Examination

Visual Examination

The women should be in lithotomy position. Look at the vulva thoroughly from mons to perineum. Inspect the labium majora from anterior to posterior commisure and the medial borders whether they appose each other or are separated, exposing the introitus. In virgins the labia are firmly apposing each other and do not get separated even with complete abduction of thighs.

Examine for injuries which may range from redness to obvious tears in the hymen by penile penetration or crescentric abrasion by forcible digital separation or tooth impression by the act of cunnilingus.

Search for evidences as hair, saliva, blood or semen transferred from the male during the sexual act—Locard's principle.

Tactile Examination

Note whether pubic hair is present or not. If present, whether there is matting or not. If matting, the matted pubic hair should be cut with scissors and air dried and packed in a clean polythene or paper envelope. If there is no matting search for loose hairs by combing with a new comb and preserve the same separately in a polythene cover. To find out whether the loose hair belongs to the victim or the accused, a few hairs must be pulled as control for comparison. Wet stains of body fluid should be collected with dry sterile gauze piece and the same preserved after being air dried. Dried stains must be scraped with scalpel or by using sterile saline soaked gauze piece or cotton swab and put in sterile test tube after being air dried. Document the injuries pertaining to the type (tear, abrasion, ecchymoses or redness), nature (colour, age, stage of healing), size and site. Trace evidence should be promptly sealed and handed over to the escort police personnel for onward transit to the biology division of forensic laboratory after due acknowledgement is obtained.

After finishing this important examination wear gloves, palpate the genitals to appreciate any subjective evidence of pain and tenderness. Examine the introitus if necessary by separating the opposing majori digitally (virgin) and examine the clitoris for its size and colour. In virgins the clitoris is small soft and slightly pigmented usually concealed under labiae but in deflorated women it becomes enlarged, dark in colour and thickened and protrudes.

Labium minora are hidden under majora in virgins, and is a pinkish, soft structure, that undergoes stretching during intercourse and becomes dark and thick after repeated sex. The injuries ranging from redness to tear can be appreciated by the MO. Below the clitoris the urethral opening and the surrounding soft mucosa should be inspected for evidence of digital or penile penetrations.

Below the urethra the vaginal outlet should be inspected along with hymenal membrane. Note whether the hymen is intact or not. If hymen is not intact, search for fresh tears and/or old tear. The free margin of the hymen should be inspected, if necessary with a magnifying lens. Note the site of the tear and document the same. The position of the tear being compared to the clock face. Coital injuries are usually present over the posterior half, whereas non-coital tears are rare and are usually seen on the anterior half of the hymen.

Fresh tear shows frank bleeding from the edges and 12 to 24 hours after the bleeding stops, the edges are swollen and edematous and bleed on touch up to 48 hours, then healing continues and complete healing occurs from 5 to 7 days after the last coitus. Once the hymen is ruptured, it is never reunited and appears as tags after repeated acts. The coital tear usually extends up to the vaginal vault which is not present in non-coital tear. There is no rigid rule to assert that the healing time of ruptured hymen is 5–7 days as it may sometimes take even 7–10 days and this depends on the severity and extent of tear and genital hygiene and health of the victim.

Below the vaginal outlet the fossa navicularis, which is situated between the posterior margin of the vaginal orifice and posterior commisure should be inspected carefully with a magnifying glass. This is the area that undergoes maximum stretch by the penile thrust and bears the impact of the act and hence sustains injury even in married women. Fossa navicularis is the free border of fourchette which is attached with the perineal body which is firm and fixed. This area is invariably neglected during examination by most MO.

Tears like minute cracks can be seen with the help of a hand lens. These tears usually heal with scar from 7 to 10 days after last coitus.

Fourchette also shows evidences of sexual assault/act ranging from redness to tears with severe bleeding especially in very young children and sometimes this may require immediate surgical intervention.

Finally the vaginal canal should be examined before vaginal swabs are to be collected, so as to avoid contamination. At least three swabs one from the fourchette, one from the vaginal canal and another from the posterior fornix must be collected and secured in sterile test tubes with proper labeling.

Deep Digital Examination

Examination of vaginal canal must be done finally with introduction of one or two fingers to assess the size of the vaginal opening to feel the rugosity of vaginal wall and further up to feel the fornices and also the state of cervix. In case of young children or virgins digital examination can be done with the help of vaginal speculum to appreciate the normal or altered structure of the vaginal wall. If there is suspected seminal fluid present, make smears over the glass slides at least two in number and allow it to be air dried and then send it for analysis and to the biology division of the forensic laboratory.

Finally the surrounding structures such as the perineam, anal and inner aspects of thigh should be examined for evidences of physical intervention as well as for dried stains of blood, semen, etc.

Thus the examination of a sexual assault victim is performed in the same manner as a gynaecological examination but differs methodically as a compassionate manner is the need of the hour and the medical officer should remember that his/her examination with interpretation of findings is absolutely necessary and vital.

OPINION

At the end of examination the doctor should conclude the following points positively before framing the opinion.

1. Whether the allegation is true or false
2. Whether the victim is virgin (unmarried) or deflorate
3. Whether there are signs of struggle or resistance
4. Whether there are signs of genital violence

Based on the above facts any one of the following can be given with your justification.

I am of opinion that there are

1. Evidences of recent sexual intercourse (genital injuries with or without general violence and detectable trace evidences)
2. Evidences of sexual intercourse but not recent (thick dark clitoris, protruding dark and thick minora, healed hymenal tears, patulous vagina, dark thick fossa navicularis)
3. No evidence of sexual intercourse (absence of genital and general violence with signs of virginity) on the victim.

    Opinion should be given within 24 hours of examination without waiting for analytical report.

CHECKLIST FOR EXAMINATION

1. Comply with the request made by investigating authority or the individual herself.

    The MO should understand, it is mandatory on her/his part that, no female victim of sexual assault should be turned away from the casualty/hospital when she complains of sexual abuse. The victim should be immediately examined. If there is any doubt/issue always consult a senior medicolegal consultant. After examination inform the jurisdiction police who will send the concerned requisition. Do not delay the examination of the victim as it interferes with the interpretation of the findings which can rule/refute the case.

2. Document the identifying information of the individual to be examined, place, time and date of examination, person accompanied or brought the individual with valid consent for examination along with two identification marks preferably on exposed parts of the body.

3. General examination starting from clothings for evidence that connect the place (gravel, grass, dirt, dry leaves, mud, etc.), evidences of forcible removal (tears, loss of hook or button) and evidences of sexual union (saliva, blood, semen, hair, etc.), examine the individual completely for assessment of physical capability to struggle, signs of scuffle and struggle and also for trace evidences such as hair, fiber, saliva, blood and semen on the body. Document and preserve all the findings carefully.

4. Meticulous genital examination methodically from external to internal for evidences of trauma, trace evidences, etc.

5. Corroborate the physical findings of general and genital examinations with the evaluated history to determine whether the incident is consistent or inconsistent with the alleged manner and time.

6. Positive analytical report is a scientific support but negative report does not rule out the alleged offence.
7. Formulate the opinion based on your physical findings as the
   (a) Victim has been exposed to sexual intercourse recently or
   (b) Exposed to sexual intercourse but not recently
   (c) Has had no sexual intercourse at all (virgin).
8. Never incorporate the word "RAPE" in the opinion.

CHECKLIST FOR EVIDENCE COLLECTION

1. Suspected stains of blood or semen on clothings. The site of stain on the cloth indicates the position of the victim.
2. Pubic hair (matter), loose hair, plucked hair, scalp hair
3. Vaginal smear and swabs
4. Blood and saliva for DNA profile.
5. Urine for drug assay.
6. Nail scrapings whenever history of assault is present.

Retrieval of the above items varies from case to case and is not necessary in cases reported after a long delay. If the victim's age is required, age should be assessed by physical, dental and radiological examination, with a separate requisition from the magistrate only and never from the police officer.

SEXUAL ASSAULT—EXAMINATION OF ACCUSED

Introduction

Though it is easy for a woman to lodge a complaint of sexual assault against a male, it is difficult to prove the same, yet much more difficult to disprove. Hence, a comprehensive examination of both victim and assailant should be immediately done to conclude or exclude the accusation. As with other clinical examination a systemic approach is essential in the examination of the accused.

Aim of the Examination

The aim is to determine:

Whether he is physically capable to perform the sexual act?

Whether there is any sign of violence on his body sustained during the scuffle/struggle at the time of occurrence?

Whether there is physical evidence which can be proof of link with victim?

Whether he is suffering from sexually transmitted diseases or any other contagious disease which is also a proof of connection with the victim, however, this STD should be treated immediately to prevent further spread.

To document all the positive and the negative findings of examination in order to frame an opinion and for future appraisal in the court of law.

Pre-requirement

A written authorization from competent police or judicial officer is mandatory. The requisition along with brief history of the events, circumstances with identifying information of the assailant are required.

Precautions

Establish the identity positively.

Written informed consent must be obtained.

Informed refusal must be obtained if he objects the physical examination.

If the accused is already under arrest or remand, consent is not mandatory, however, it is advisable to get written consent to avoid unwanted allegations.

Procedure of Examination

After fulfilling the initial formalities first document the identifying information as follows:

Time, date and place of examination.

Identification of requesting authority with his designation, jurisdiction, reference/crime number, date.

Identification of the escort police with his number, rank and name.

Identifying information of the accused such as name, father's name, age, sex, address, occupation, marital status, two identification marks preferably on exposed parts of the body. The above information has to be documented for the purpose of identification at a later stage even after years.

History Evaluation

History relating to the complaint leveled against him by the female should be elicited in detail but invariably the accused person always denies the accusation.

Personal History

Social status of the victim, acquaintance with the victim, recent illness (medical history), recent surgery, if any, habits such as smoking, alcohol, drugs, etc.

Medical History

Particular attention should be given to nervous disorders, metabolic disorders and medication must be recorded.

Surgical and Traumatic History

Surgery involving the perineal region, history of fall into manhole or any traumatic injury involving the genitals, head, and spinal column should be elicited.

Sexual History

Sexual contact before and after the present incident.

Details of the crime should be elicited to corroborate with the victim's statement to plan the investigation and also to retrieve trace evidences.

General Examination

To assess the physical ability to overpower the victim, physical features such as height, weight, shoulder, chest and abdominal girth must be measured. To assess the age if accused claims as minor, hair growth over the pubis, axilla, face and scalp, dental pattern and to assess the bone maturation, radiological assessment of shoulder, elbow, wrist, pelvis, ankle and knee joint are to be taken. Assess the general health and rule out certain systemic diseases which potentially interferes with sexual capability. Pulse, BP, respiratory rate and other vital parameters are to be recorded. Search for evidence of physical injuries ranging from scratches, contusion, lip, tear, etc. as signs of struggle along with tear, defect or loss of button or zip in the shirt and pant. Examine for the presence of trace evidences as mud, dirt, sand, grass, fiber, hair, blood or salivary stain and the undergarment for blood or seminal stain. The trace evidences must be collected carefully after documenting properly and forwarded safely for analysis.

Genital Examination

This should be done in a systematic manner as follows.

Inspection of the external genital organs for developmental defects and localized diseases which can obviously interfere with the sexual act, and signs of traumatic lesions which could have been sustained during the alleged sexual assault or signs of surgical intervention in the past and the structural and functional integrity of the testes.

First note the pubic hair, if it is matted, it should be cut; air dried and kept in a paper envelope for analysis. If there is no matting, look for foreign hair by gentle combing which may belong to him or to the female. If loose hairs are detected collect them, then a few hairs must be pulled out for control sample and they should be preserved separately in paper envelope. Examine for blood or seminal stains over the penis, scrotum and inner aspects of thighs and also for injuries such as abrasion, contusion and frenular tear. Examine the prepuce for cracks if uncircumcised, and check whether it is retractable or not. Look for smegma under the prepuce and state of the frenulum which is usually torn during the first act of coitus. Presence of smegma suggests that there is no sexual intercourse in the preceeding 24 hours and absence of smegma may be due to being wiped away during intercourse or washed off during bath. Once smegma is wiped or washed off it will take 24 hours to recollect.

The penile shaft is 7.5–10 cm long in flaccid state and the circumference is 3–5 cm. The glans penis is covered by prepucial skin in uncircumcised persons and the urethra opens at the tip of the glans. The size of the penis does not correlate with the stature and muscularity of the individual. Developmental defect such as micropenis, double penis, hypo and epispadiasis necessarily interfere with the physical ability of the individual to perform sexual act. Evidences of sexually transmitted diseases which causes temporary impotence like gonorrhoea, soft and hard chancre, lymphoma and lymphadenitis should be looked for. The scrotal sac should be examined for traumatic or surgical scar (vasectomy) and the testes for huge hydrocoele, huge hernia and elephantiasis which also interfere with sexual intercourse.

For various causes of impotence in male refer to questions and answers at the end of this chapter.

The functional integrity can be tested by penile erection (ask the accused to hold the penis in his left hand with slight force with to and fro stroke with the prepuce over the glans or with the glans alone if circumcised, something sort of masturbation) or by eliciting pubo-scrotal reflex (gentle stroke over inner aspect of upper third of thigh with the pointed end of knee—hammer or with a ear bud). The testicle moves upward in the scrotal sac of the side where the stroke is applied. This indicates intact and integrated nerve supply.

Next, look for injuries which are likely to result from forcible sexual intercourse such as tearing of fraenum or bruising of glans. Search for injuries sustained during the struggle caused by the victim such as abrasion, contusion, redness, and tenderness over the lower abdomen, scrotum and thighs.

Look for blood stains, vaginal discharge or seminal stains, etc. if the assailant had not washed or bathed since the act. The vaginal epithelium adherent to the glans penis in recent vaginal penetration can be collected by using a filter paper preserved after getting air dried, for analysis.

If blood and/or seminal stains are detected from the clothings or genitalia of the victim, blood from the accused has to be collected for grouping, DNA typing and also saliva to find out his secretor state.

If the accused claims as impotent, he should be referred to an urologist to rule out the organic cause of impotence since law considers that every man is presumed to be potent until the contrary is proved.

In short, the purpose of the examination of accused person is to find out:

1. Whether he is capable of performing sexual intercourse?
2. Whether there is any subjective evidence of struggle?
3. Whether there is any objective evidence of linkage between him and the victim?

The examination of the accused is rarely done immediately as he is brought for examination after a delay of a few days to even a few weeks.

Evidence Collection

Determination of trace evidence collection from the accused person depends upon the following factors:

1. Time lapsed after the alleged sexual act.
2. Discovery of blood, seminal, salivary-stain, foreign pubic hair, or epithelial debris under the nails from the victim.
3. Evidence of sexually transmitted disease.
4. Pregnancy

In Cases Where the Accused is Brought Immediately

Materials to be Retrieved

1. Undergarments for detection of blood, seminal or vaginal discharge after documentation in the register about physical state, and exact portion of the undergarment. If stains are wet get it air dried, then pack carefully in paper envelopes avoiding folding over the stained area.

2. Hair: Pubic hair—matted tuft—packed after air drying.

Loose hair—preserved separately with the comb.

Plucked hair—preserve separately.

Pulled out scalp hair—for DNA typing.

3. Smears taken from penile shaft and glans with filter paper for detection of vaginal epithelium by Lugol iodine test.

In Cases of Delayed Examination Usually 24 hours After the Alleged Sexual Act

1. Blood for grouping and DNA typing
2. Saliva to determine his secretor state.

Blood and saliva can be collected with sterile dry gauze piece packed after air drying.

In addition to this if the accused is found intoxicated, blood and urine should be collected appropriately for alcohol estimation/drug assay.

Invariably on many occasions the investigating authorities ask for collection of semen from the accused person. It must be emphasized that there is no need to collect semen in all cases of sexual assault in order to find out the seminal group. This can be substituted with collection of blood and saliva scientifically.

It has been proved that 80% of the population are secretors in whom the group specific substance is the same in all the body fluids including semen.

Suppose the blood and saliva belong to the same group, then the seminal fluid also belongs to that same group.

Seminal collection is warranted on following occasions

- If the accused is a non-secretor
- In case of gang rape
- In case where the victim and the accused have the same blood group.
- If the victim is pregnant and the accused claims he is sterile.

No evidence need to be collected where there is a considerable delay in reporting and examination.

One should always bear in mind that positive analytical reports alone are not proof of connection between the victim and accused, since sexual intercourse can be committed without leaving any trace in either partner.

Conclusion

At the end of the examination it has to be concluded about the physical capability of the accused to perform sexual intercourse. It is a fact that every man is presumed to be potent but there are certain organic functional disorders that may render a man incapable of having sexual connection. During the course of general and specific examination, one can easily detect obvious anatomical defects, diseases, post-traumatic or surgical complications that are the virtual causes of physical impotence. However, it is difficult to assess the psychological component of potency. In most cases a male with normally developed genital organs without having any obvious diseases to interfere with his physique, cannot be declared as potent, since sex is initiated by sensory stimulus which varies from individual to individual and also from time to time in the same individual. Since there is no definite procedure or parameter to measure this psychological component, opinion on potency cannot be given straightaway as in the case of obvious organic diseases. Hence the opinion should be given indirectly in double negative phrases. The positive analytical report is a proof of union having corroborative value only, since the negative report does not rule out the presence of a sexual connection.

Opinion is Always Given As

I am of the opinion that there is "nothing to suggest that the individual I have examined, is incapable of performing sexual intercourse".

EVALUATORY QUESTIONS

1. **What is rape?**

   Rape is a legal term, not a medical diagnosis. The word *rape* is derived from a Latin word "Rapere" meaning of which is steal or snatch. Legal concept of rape is different from medical concept of sexual intercourse. Rape can be committed by penetration of penis into the vulva with or without erection, with or without ejaculation, with a woman against her will or without her consent, or her consent obtained by force, fraud or by fear of harm or threat of death to her or her loved one, or with consent with a girl under 18 years or in a state of intoxication or unconsciousness.

   The medical concept is sexual intercourse is very different from the legal definition of rape.

2. **Which section of IPC defines rape?**

   Rape is defined under Section 375 of Indian Penal Code as a man is said to commit *rape* when he has sexual intercourse with a woman under circumstances falling under any of the following six categories:

   1. Against her will
   2. Without her consent
   3. With her consent, when her consent has been obtained by putting her or any other person in whom she is interested in fear of death or hurt.
   4. With her consent, when the man knows that he is not her husband and that her consent is given because she believes that he is the man to whom she is or believes herself to be lawfully married.
   5. With her consent when at the time of giving such consent, by reason of unsoundness of mind or due to intoxication or by the administration of any drug/stupefying substance, etc. to her personally or through another person. She is unable to understand the nature and consequences of the act to which she gives consent.
   6. With or without her consent when she is under 18 years of age.

   Exception: Sexual intercourse by a man with his wife when the wife is not being under fifteen years of age is not rape.

3. **What are the patterns of rape?**

The different patterns of rape are:
1. Rape by a known person (constructive rape)
2. Rape by unknown (stranger rape)
3. Date rape—occurs in dating couples
4. Mate rape—compulsive sex with rapist
5. Marital rape—wife raped by husband
6. Partner rape—co-habitation
7. Statutory rape—sex with a girl under 16 years
8. Spite rape—sexual connection so as to blackmail or to avenge on the victim
9. Feigned rape—pretending to have been raped
10. Custodial rape

4. **Name section of the IPC to award punishment for rape.**

Section 376 IPC describes punishment for rape as follows: Whoever except in the cases provided for by subsection commits rape shall be punished with imprisonment of either description for a term which shall not be less than 7 years but which may be for life or for a term which may extend to 10 years and shall also be liable to fine unless the woman raped is his own wife and is not under 12 years of age in which case he shall be punished with imprisonment of either for a term which may extend to 2 years or fine or with both.

Subsection 2:

(a) Police officer commits rape
    1. Within his station limit
    2. Within the premises of any other police station
    3. A woman in his or his subordinate custody

(b) A public servant misusing his official position and power
(c) Official of a jail, remand home or institution for destitute women and children
(d) Official of a hospital
(e) Rape on a pregnant woman
(f) Rape on a girl under 12 years
(g) Gang rape

Shall be punished with rigorous imprisonment for a term which shall not be less than 10 years but which may be for life and shall also be liable for fine.

5. **What is unlawful sexual offence not amounting to rape?**

Sexual intercourse by a man with a woman under circumstances which do not fall under any of the criteria described in Section 375 IPC is known as "unlawful sexual intercourse but not amounting to rape" and this is also punishable under 376 A–D according to varying circumstances.

Marital rape: Intercourse by a man with his wife under a degree of separation or customary separation is punishable under Section 376A IPC for a term which may extend to two years also liable to fine.

376B: A public servant takes advantage of his official position and induces or seduces a woman in his custody or under the custody of his subordinate to have sexual intercourse with him shall be punished with imprisonment for a term which may extend to five years and shall also be liable to fine.

376C: A prison or remand home official induces or seduces a woman under his custody by misusing his official position to have a sexual connection with him, shall be punished with imprisonment for a term which may extend to five years and shall also be liable to fine.

376D: Intercourse by any member of the management or staff of a hospital with any woman in that hospital shall be punished with imprisonment for a term which may extend to five years and also be liable to fine.

Section 509 IPC: Word, gesture or act intended to insult the modesty of a woman is punishable with imprisonment for a term which may extend to one year or with fine or with both.

6. **What do you mean by unnatural sexual offences and what is the punishment for unnatural sexual offences?**

Intercourse against the order of nature with any man, woman or animal is known as unnatural sexual offences.

For example, buccal coitus, anal intercourse, bestiality

377 IPC is the punishment section for unnatural sexual offences punishable with imprisonment for life or for a term which may extend to ten years and shall also be liable to fine.

7. **What is meant by statutory rape?**

Statutory rape denotes the sexual intercourse by a man with a woman under the age of 16 even with her consent.

8. **What are the ages which have medicolegal importance in relation to sexual offences?**

Age 12: Under Section 376 IPC whoever commits the offence of rape is punishable with imprisonment not less than 7 years and may extend up to 10 years. But if the age of the victim is below 12 years, the accused has to be punished with rigorous punishment not less than 10 years, may even be sentenced for life imprisonment, and if the girl is married, the husband is also punishable in the same manner.

Age 15: There is an exception under Section 375 that the husband of a married girl whose age is 15 years is not punishable but if the age is less than 15 he is liable to be punished up to 2 years only.

Age 16: This is the age in which the woman acquires the right to select her partner. Having sexual intercourse with her consent beyond this age is not considered rape but if she is below 16, her consent is not at all valid.

Age 18: According to Section 372 IPC selling or letting to hire or otherwise disposal of any woman under 18 years is liable for punishment up to 10 years and the same is applicable for letting a woman with a person not united by marriage, neither legally nor accepted by the society and customs for intercourse is also liable to be punished up to 10 years for "illicit intercourse" if the girl is below 18 years.

As per 373 IPC buying or hiring or obtaining possession of a girl under 18 years for the purpose of prostitution or illicit intercourse is liable for punishment up to 10 years.

9. **What is impotence?**

   Impotence is defined as the inability to achieve or to maintain the erectile function of penis and to perform successful coitus.

10. **What are the types of impotence?**

    There are two types of impotence.
    1. Primary impotence: Sexual intercourse has never been performed successfully.
    2. Secondary impotence: Inability to have successful coitus following at least one successful coital act.
    3. Conditional impotence: Insufficient erection during the initial phase of the sexual act usually achieved by manual stimulation or fellatio or resistance of the victim.

11. **What are the causes of impotence in male (erectile dysfunction)?**

    1. Physiological
    2. Psychological
    3. Organic
    4. Drug induced/abused.

12. **What is the angle of erected penis?**

    The angle of erected penis is 25° to 35° without any support.

13. **What is the difference between impotency and sterility?**

    Impotency denotes the inability to perform successful intercourse, whereas sterility denotes the inability to impregnate.

Thanatology

Section 2

6   Skeletal Remains—Examination

INTRODUCTION

Bones are the living connective tissue which is composed of protein (collagen) and mineral (hydroxyapatite). The skeleton forms the framework giving attachment to the soft tissues, protects the vital organs, locomotion by giving attachment to muscles, tendons and ligaments. Apart from these physical functions bones are the sites of storage of fats and minerals and synthesis of blood cells (haemopoiesis). Hence bones are the dynamic tissue which undergoes growth during development, responding to day to day stress and strain and reactivation to repair the fracture site.

Why Study Bones?

As like other body tissues and organs, the bones also ceased to function after death and undergo decay. But the decaying process in the bones occurs more slowly than the soft tissues; hence the bones are the most lasting evidence of human existence. The skeleton is just like a horoscope which recollects the past, reveals the present and the future can also be predicted with the time and date of birth of an individual. Like that of a horoscope bones also reflect the biological identity of the individual determined genetically and also the evidence of employment, illness, injury sustained and suffered during life of that individual. Because of the above mentioned reasons examination of bone is not only mandatory but also the only evidence of a missing person available in medicolegal death investigation, many a times. Thus the inference of this examination can be compared and corroborated with the biological and physical characters of the alleged missing/deceased either to confirm or to exclude the identity.

In forensic practice autopsies are being carried out on fresh bodies regularly and fleshed decomposed bodies occasionally. At times exhumation and examination of skeletal remains also required to assist the medicolegal death investigation. Establishing the personal identity is mandatory to proceed further into the death investigation to establish manner, time and cause and also to bring a strong alibi. Usually the dead bodies of criminal death are being disposed in places not to be easily detected and identified; by the time of detection nothing could be visualized except the skeleton. Hence the knowledge of skeletal remains examination is most important for doctors to establish identity and to assist the investigators in establishing the truth beyond any doubt.

How to Retrieve Bones?

Though all the bones of the human skeleton are useful, the bones which bear the most important findings to establish the identity of an individual should be selected for examination. Based on this fact, priority is given to skull or cranium, pelvis, femur, tibia, humerus, radius and scapula.

Each bone speaks about the genetically determined facts of its owner such as age, sex, stature and ethnicity (biological profile) and also about the effects of employment, illness, injury faced by the individual (idiosyncratic profile). Before determining the above traits of personal identification, it is mandatory and preliminary to know whether the available bone belongs to human or not (species identification). After fixing the personal identity the time elapsed after death can be ascertained by decaying changes of the bone.

The ultimate purpose of examination of skeletal remains is to answer the following points on each bone available.

Is the bone human? (Species identification)   (Origin)

If human

1. Does it belong to a male or female?   (Sex)
2. What could be the age at death?   (Age)
3. What could be the height at death?   (Stature)
4. Which part of the world he/she belongs?   (Race)
5. How long ago death could have occurred?   (Time since death)
6. What could be the cause of death?   (Cause of death)
7. What could be the manner of death?   (Etiology of death)
8. Is there any peculiar feature due to occupation, disease or trauma not connected to the cause of death or unusual features such as metopism, tarus mandibularis, etc.?
9. When two or more than two bones are available, is it mandatory to find out whether they belong to the same or different individual (comminglingness)?

Species Identification

To find out the species of a bone three methods are useful which depends upon the nature of the available bone. They are visual examination, microscopic examination and immunological examination.

Visual Examination

When the bone is full and intact, a gross appearance will speak about its origin. The size and shape of a bone determined by form and functional differences between the animal and human.

For example, the forelimb bones in animals (pronograde and quadruped) are more massive and stronger to perform fast running and also to bear the weight of the anterior half of the body and head, whereas their counterparts in human (orthograde and biped) are modified to perform useful functions. This is applicable to all the bones; hence knowledge of comparison anatomy is more useful in determining the origin. Cortex of long bone in human is 1/4 of total diameter, whereas in other mammals 1/3 of cut section.

Origin: It is merely a comparison of size and shape of the bone with animals (comparison anatomy) (Figs 6.1 and 6.2).

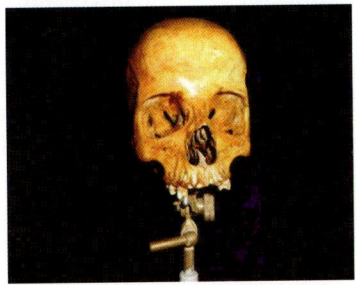

Fig. 6.1: Human

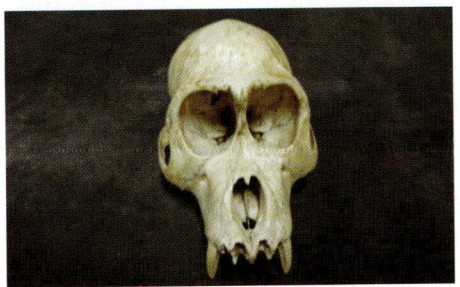

Fig. 6.2: Monkey

Histological Examination

If incomplete and broken bones or small bones alone is given, visual examination is no way useful. During that occasion microscopic examination of a thin bone section is useful to differentiate human from animal. The human bone can be identified by the lamellae with well developed haversian system, whereas the animal bone with lamellar pattern and ill developed haversian canals. In humans, osteons are scattered. Whereas in animals, they are lined up in rows like a stack of bricks.

Immunological Examination

When the available bone is very small, irregular or fragmented, then prepare a solution with weak hydrochloric acid or ammonia and this solution that contains bone protein is the antigen. When this antigen is treated with specific antibody, antigen–antibody reaction occurs with precipitation. If the test solution from the bone reacts with antibody of human, it is of human origin. If it does not react, it is negative for human antibody and hence it is not of human origin.

Sex Identification

Once the bone is identified as human bone, the next step is to find out whether it belongs to male or female. If sex of the bone is established, the search area will be reduced to 50% because one sex of the population can be excluded. Sex of a bone can be determined by structural and functional variations.

In general men are stronger, larger and masculine and women are smaller, lighter and feminine. These general characters are implied upon the bones also. Hence the bones of males are larger, longer and thicker, whereas the female bones are gracile, smaller and smoother. These general characteristics are applicable to all bones but better visualised only after puberty remarkably.

The functional difference between male and female bone is found classically in pelvis since the female pelvis is designed for child birth by nature. All these sexual dimorphism will be discussed with individual bones. The best bone of human skeleton to determine sex is pelvis (95% accuracy), next skull (90% accuracy) and long bones (80% accuracy). Pelvis + Skull = 98%, Pelvis + Long bones = 98%.

Age Determination

The next important question is the age of the person when he or she died (period of survival after birth). The basic concept in determination of age from examination of bone is the sequential changes that occur in bones as a person ages.

To understand how to estimate the age from bone one must understand how the skeleton is formed and what are the changes that occur in the bones periodically as the person grows from childhood and progressively to adulthood. Like the soft tissues and organs the bones also develop at a different rate at different age in a fairly regular sequence. Though all bones undergo age changes, the best and reliable are the limb bones and teeth eruption from childhood to adulthood. When full growth is attained gradual reduction in bone density occurs from 5th decade onwards. Post-adult age can be reliably estimated with changing morphology over the symphysial face of pubis, iliac articular surface and sutural closure of skull.

Calcification of sternal end of ribs especially the 4th rib, laryngeal and thyroid cartilage and fusion of manubrium with the mesosternum are also useful parameters to assess the age after 4th decade of life. In general the accuracy of the skeletal age estimate becomes wider as the person grows older since the developmental changes over the bone is more distinct in young, whereas the degeneration changes are more difficult and less distinct hence the accuracy rate is inversely proportionate with advancing age.

Stature Calculation

Stature is one of the important biological characteristics which can be estimated from the long bones more consistently because of their contribution to the total stature of an individual. The most reliable bone to determine the height is the femur followed by tibia, humerus and radius. Maximum length of the bone should be measured with Hepburn osteometric board (not by measuring with tapes or calibers) and then calculate the stature with a mathematical formula devised by

1. Trotter and Gleser
2. Karl Pearson

For Indians there has not been any proper research done satisfactorily, but mathematical calculations with multiplication factors for each long bone is devised by their percentage contribution to the total stature which was devised by Topinard as humerus 20%, tibia 22%, femur 27% and vertebral column 33% with an allowance of 3–4 cm for soft tissues.

Race Determination

The question of race arises in certain occasions where people from different parts of the world have been involved in an air crash or bomb blast or train accident or other natural calamities. Under the above circumstances identification of the victims become crucial to claim the monetary and other benefits by the relatives of the deceased.

Though racial characters are genetically determined it is modified by cultural practices also. Race of an individual can be mostly determined by facial skeleton and of course from long bones also. Firstly let us determine the above said biological profile of the individual from the appropriate bones.

SEX DETERMINATION BY INDIVIDUAL BONES

Apart from the general differences between male and female bones specific sexual dimorphism can be studied by the functional modification and evolutionary adaptation of female pelvis as parturition is the most important function. Because of these functional differences pelvic bone is the first best part of skeleton that provides the most accurate and reliable result for sex determination, and next is the skull and long bones are the last.

Sex Determination From Pelvis

Pelvis alone gives 95% accuracy in sex determination.

Pelvis consists of two important bones articulating posteriorly with sacrum and anteriorly both pubic bones meet at the symphysis. Each innominate bone is composed of three parts, i.e. ilium, ischium, and pubis which fuse together after puberty. The following are the morphologic and morphometric differences which are useful to determine the exact sex of the pelvis.

Morphologic (Visual) Sex Traits

Table 6.1: Morphologic sex traits—pelvis

		Male	*Female*
1.	General shape	Long and narrow like a funnel	Short and broad like a bowl
2.	Pelvic inlet	Heart shaped	Oval shaped
3.	Sacral promontory	Prominent	Smooth
4.	Iliac crest	Hard and rough	Smooth
5.	Muscle markings	Rough and rugged	Smooth
6.	Ischial tuberosity	Rough and inverted	Thin and everted
7.	Acetabulum	Big and facing outwards (Fig. 6.7) (diameter 52 mm)	Small, facing forwards and out (Fig. 6.8) (diameter 46 mm)
8.	Greater sciatic notch	Narrow and deep(< 58°) (Fig. 6.5) Accommodate the tip of thumb tightly without space for wriggling	Wide and shallow(>50°) (Fig. 6.6) Allows the thumb to wriggle freely
9.	Preauricular sulcus	Least or not prominent	Prominent
10.	Postauricular sulcus	Least or not prominent	Prominent
11.	Obturator foramen	Oval in shape	Triangular in shape
12.	Subpubic angle	Acute < 90° (Fig. 6.3) Angle between index and middle finger approximately fits	Obtuse > 90° (Fig. 6.4) Angle between thumb and index finger approximately fits
13.	Body of pubis	Small and triangular	Big and rectangular
14.	Ventral ramus	Not prominent	More prominent
15.	Subpubic concavity	Not prominent	More prominent
16.	Sacrum	Narrow and long	Broad and short
17.	Sacral curvature	Uniform concavity above downwards	Vertical in the upper part, deep concavity in the middle with forward projection at the end (curve of carus)
18.	Articular surface	Long and wide	Short and narrow
19.	Ischial tuberosity	Everted	Inverted
20.	Ischio pubic ramus	Straight/convex	Always concave

Subpubic Angle

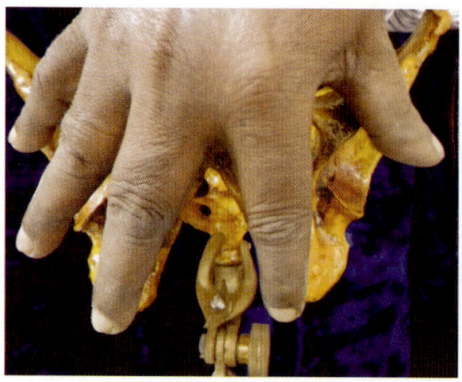

Fig. 6.3: Male pelvis—acute

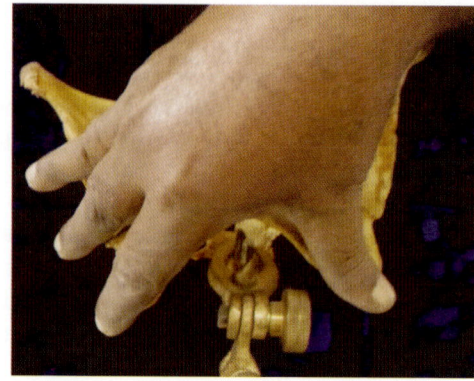

Fig. 6.4: Female pelvis—Obtuse

Greater Sciatic Notch

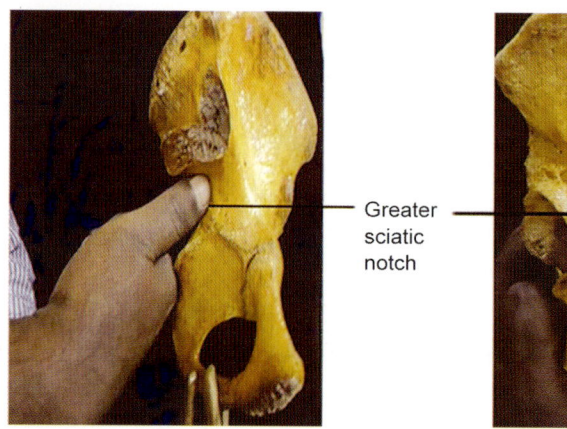

Greater sciatic notch

Fig. 6.5: Greater sciatic notch

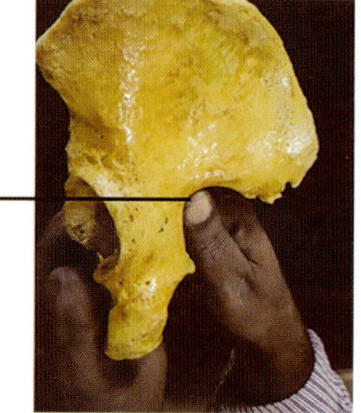

Fig. 6.6: Greater sciatic notch

Acetabulum

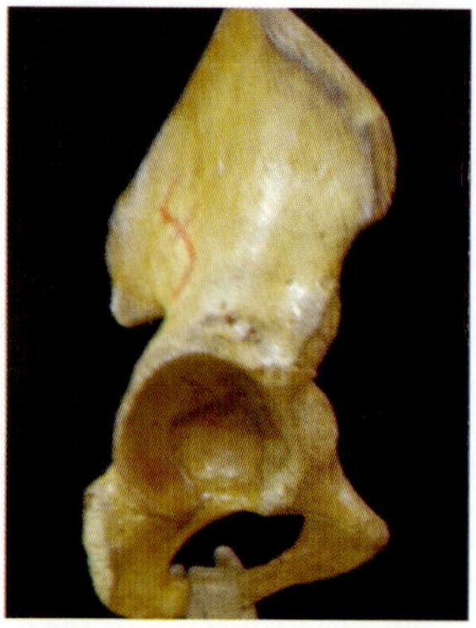

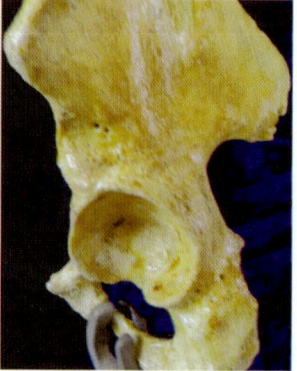

Fig. 6.7: Male pelvis—deep

Fig. 6.8: Female pelvis—shallow

Pelvimetry

1. Sciatic Index

The ratio between the width and depth of the sciatic notch.

$$\text{Sciatic index} = \frac{\text{Width of sciatic notch}}{\text{Depth of sciatic notch}} \times 100$$

Male = 4 – 5, Female = 5 – 6

2. Ischiopubic Index

The ratio between the length of the pubis and length of the ischium.

$$\text{Ischiopubic index} = \frac{\text{Length of pubis}}{\text{Length of ischium}} \times 100$$

Male ≤ 90,   Female ≥ 94

3. Sacral Index (SI)

The ratio between the breadth and anterior length of the sacrum

$$\text{SI} = \frac{\text{Breadth of sacrum (body with alae)}}{\text{Anterior length of sacrum}} \times 100$$

Male ≤ 122,   Female ≥ 116

4. Corporobasal Index (CBI)

The ratio between the breadth of body of first sacral vertebra and breadth of base of sacrum including alae.

$$\text{CBI} = \frac{\text{Breadth of body}}{\text{Breadth of base}} \times 100$$

Male ≥ 45,   Female ≤ 40

5. Base Wing Index (BWI)

The ratio between the transverse diameter of body of first sacral vertebra and transverse width of ala on one side.

$$\text{BWI} = \frac{\text{Transverse diameter of one ala}}{\text{Transverse diameter of body}} \times 100$$

Male = 65,   Female = 75

Sex Determination From Skull

Next to the pelvis skull is the most useful bone to determine the sex.

Morphological Sex Traits

Table 6.2: Morphological sex traits—skull

		Male	Female
General			
1.	Size	Large	Small
2.	Weight	Heavy	Light
3.	Surface	Rough	Smooth
4.	Cranial cavity	More capacious	Less capacious
Facial (Figs 6.9 and 6.10)			
5.	Forehead contour	Sloping upwards and backwards	Vertical
6.	Supraorbital ridge	More prominent	Less prominent or smooth
7.	Shape of the orbit	Square	Round/oval
8.	Superolateral orbital rim	Rounded	Sharp
9.	Frontonasal junction	Deep	Shallow
10.	Nasal opening	High and narrow	Low and broad
11.	Zygomatic arch	Expanded	Compressed
Lateral view (Figs 6.11 and 6.12)			
12.	Mastoid process	Big, broad, blunt Approximately equal to the tip of thumb	Small, short and sharp Approximately equal to the tip of little finger
13.	Supramastoid crest	Prominent	Smooth
Posterior view (Figs 6.13 and 6.14)			
14.	Occipital protruberance	Prominent, protruding	Smooth and flat
15.	Nuchal Lines	Rough	Smooth
Basal view (Figs 6.15 and 6.16)			
16.	Foramen magnum	Large and long	Small and round
17.	Occipital condyles	Broad and short	Narrow and long
18.	Digastric groove	Deep	Shallow
19.	Hard palate	Large and deep	Small and shallow
Mandible			
20.	Symphyseal height	Greater	Lesser
21.	Chin	Square	Rounded
22.	Ascending ramus	Broad	Narrow
23.	Gonial angle	Everted	Inverted

Frontal view

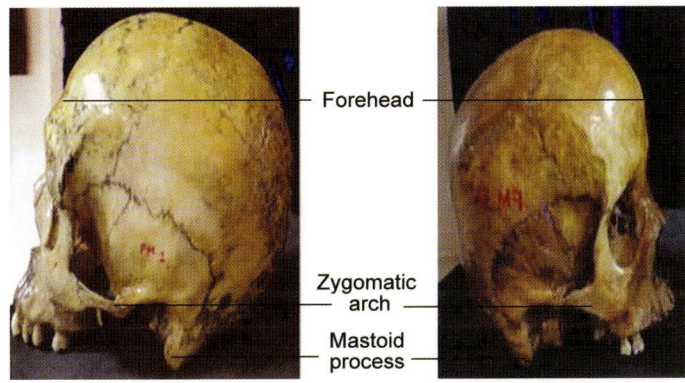

Forehead
Supraorbital ridge
Frontonasal junction
Orbit

Nasal opening

Fig. 6.9   Fig. 6.10

Lateral view

Forehead

Zygomatic arch

Mastoid process

Fig. 6.11   Fig. 6.12

Posterior view

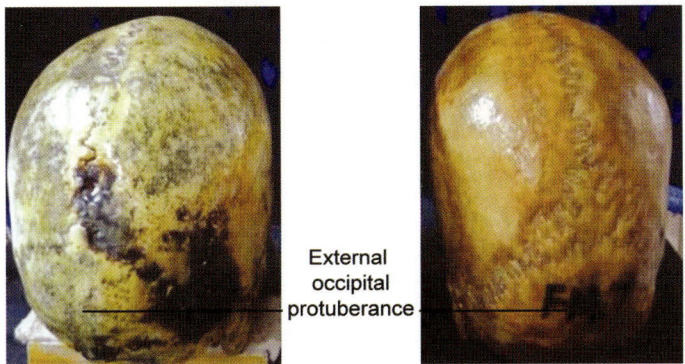

External occipital protuberance

Fig. 6.13   Fig. 6.14

Basal view

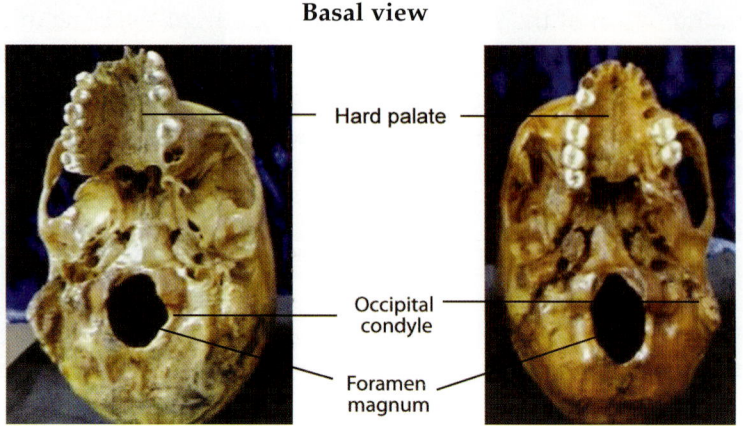

Hard palate

Occipital condyle

Foramen magnum

Fig. 6.15   Fig. 6.16

Sex Determination from Long Bones

General Characters

Male bones are longer, stronger and heavier than the female counterparts. The bones which are more useful in determining the sex are the humerus, femur, and ulna. Apart from the general characters, sex determination can be done by visual examination and morphometric methods.

Femur

Femur is the most useful of all the long bones of humans, since it is the longest, strongest and heaviest bone bearing all of the body weight during walking, standing and running.

		Male	*Female*
1.	Maximum length	> 459 mm	< 426 mm
2.	Femoral head vertical diameter	> 45 mm	< 41 mm
3.	Lower end bicondylar width	> 78 mm	< 72 mm
4.	Shaft angulation with condyles	80°	75°

When the femur is held vertically so that both condyles are resting on the surface, the shaft inclines outward more in female than male.

Humerus

		Male	*Female*
1.	Length	326 mm	298 mm
2.	Head		
	a. Vertical diameter	> 46 mm	< 45 mm
	b. Transverse diameter	> 42 mm	< 41 mm

Ulna

Sigmoid notch is usually seen in male and not in female.

Medullary Index

The ratio between the width of the medulla and total width of the bone in cross section.

All the long bones are provided with cortex and medulla. The weight of the bone depends upon the cortex. As the medullary portion in female is more, the bones of the females are lighter and gracile.

Medicolegal Importance

Medullary index is useful in sex determination in long bone such as femur, ulna and radius.

Sternum

	Male	*Female*
Total length (manubrium + body)	>140 mm	<131 mm
Manubrium corpus (sternal) index	41 mm	54 m

$$\text{Sternal index} = \frac{\text{Length of manubrium}}{\text{Length of body (mesosternum)}} \times 100$$

In general the body of sternum in males is more than twice the length of manubrium while in females it is less than twice the length of manubrium, i.e. manubrium length in females is greater than half the length of body of the sternum.

Scapula

Apart from the morphological characters of male and female bones, certain dimensions are useful to differentiate male and female scapula bones. Maximum length (between superior and inferior angles) and maximum breadth (from base of spine to glenoid cavity) are useful in sex assessment from scapula.

	Male	*Female*
Maximum length	158 mm	130 mm
Maximum breadth	100 mm	90 mm

Clavicle

Male clavicles are larger and stronger as they reflect the broader shoulders in males than the females.

	Male	*Female*
Length	> 150 mm	< 130 mm
Midshaft circumference	> 35 mm	< 30 mm

Sacrum

As the female pelvis is broader and shorter than the male pelvis, the sacrum which is articulating with the iliac bones on both sides are also broad and short with uniform concavity over the pelvic surface. Two indices are useful morphometric methods to determine the sex from sacrum.

1. **Corporobasal Index**

   Width of the body (corpus) of first sacral vertebra divided with width of base of Ist sacral vertebra (basal part of sacrum) including the ala on either sides which articulates with ilium.

   $$\text{Corporobasal index} = \frac{\text{Width of body of Ist sacral vertebra}}{\text{Width of base of sacrum}} \times 100$$

   In Males = 45,   Females = 40

2. **Base Wing Index**

   The transverse diameter of body of Ist sacral vertebral and transverse width of one ala (wing) are measured and the ratio is expressed as basal wing index.

   $$\text{Basal wing index} = \frac{\text{Width of the wing}}{\text{Width of the base}} \times 100$$

   In Males = 65,   Females = 75

From the above detailed study it is understood that the only functional difference between the male and female skeleton is well marked in pelvis as the female pelvis is designed for child birth. Hence the best bone to determine sex from human skeleton is the pelvis.

Since none of the abovementioned methods of determining sex from single bones is not easy and may yield false result. Examination of two or more bones is always advisable. When nothing is ascertained, the new technique of detecting Y chromosome by fluorescence test can be used with a special stain *quinacrine mustard* and presence of male chromosome—Y chromosome can be viewed under a fluorescence microscope in male bones.

AGE DETERMINATION BY INDIVIDUAL BONES

After ascertaining the sex, next is the age at death (that is, how old a person was when he/she died) which must be ascertained from bones. Determination of age from the bones is based on the periodical changes that occur to everyone at specific times in sequential pattern during active growth phase and wear and tear changes which affect the bones after their growth ceased. For better understanding how the age of skeleton is determined, one must know how the skeleton is formed. All the 206 bones of the adult human skeleton develops from 806 ossification centres. During development, the 806 falls to 450 centres at birth with 300 separate bones which in turn form the 206 bones of adults. All these bones do not form or grow simultaneously but grow in pieces by fusion of these ossification centres at different time in relation to growth at almost regular sequence. However, age determination from skeletal remains invokes certain bones of the skeleton such as skull, pelvis, long bones and scapula.

Age Determination from Skull

Dental Eruption

Age determination from cranium: There are certain age indicators in the skull which can yield age in narrow range on young individual and broad range (in decades) in older individual. The first age indicator is the dental pattern for which the tooth and alveolar sockets must be counted over the maxilla and apply the dental eruption formula to determine the age. For example, when the second molar is erupted and the third molar not erupted (only 7 teeth in each quadrant) then the age is above 12 years and if the third molar is also erupted then the age is above 17 years.

Sutural Fusion

The second important age indicator from the skull is the suture. The sutures are the immovable joints between the bones of the skull. These sutures are easily recognizable in the skulls of young adults but obliterates gradually with the increasing age and all these sutures iron out after 80 years.

This sutural changes with the process of ageing are the basis for determining age of individuals from the skull sutures. In this subsutural metamorphosis, five (0–4) stages have been recognised from open suture to complete sutural closure.

    0 No closure   1 Slight closure   2 Moderate closure

    3 Advance closure   4 Complete obliteration

Basal Suture

Sphenooccipital suture is situated over the base of skull between the basal part of occipital and posterior part of sphenoid bones. These two bones are connected by hyaline cartilage during the younger age which is ultimately replaced by bone between 18 and 20 years of age.

Medicolegal Significance

If the suture is fused, the skull bone belongs to a person above 18 years and if it is not fused, it indicates that the person is below 20 years.

Vault Sutures

There are three important vault sutures which are connecting the frontal, parietal and occipital bones of the cranial vault which have significance in determining the age.

A suture is a fibrous joint where the edges of the adjacent bones articulate with one another, existing only in the skull which are immovable. The margin of each bone is covered by a layer of osteogenic cells and fibrous tissue which are with the corresponding layer of periosteum over the non-articular surface of each bone. The fibrous layers of the internal and external periostea of adjacent bones form the chief band of union between the bones. In the young, the bones expand by growth at the suture. But the process of ossification continues even beyond the complete growth but at a very slow rate and hence the sutural lines gradually obliterate. This process of sutural fusion completes first over the interior of the skull (endocranial) by the age of 25 years after which the sutures over the external surface (exocranial) undergo fusion at varying ages up to 70–80 years and beyond 80 all the sutures become indistinct and the whole skull becomes smooth.

To appreciate the sutural fusion over the endocranial aspect a good source of light must be focused through the foramen magnum. If the sutures are distinctly visible, it indicates the age is below 25 years and if no suture is distinctly seen, it indicates the age is above 25 years.

When the sutures are fused over the endocranium next the exocranial sutures should be examined. First, the *sagittal suture* which lies between the parietal bones on either side running anteroposteriorly from bregma to lambda. This suture must be divided into three segments by two imaginatory transverse lines.

The posterior 1/3rd of the suture fuses first between 30 and 40 years, next the anterior 1/3rd between 40 and 50 years and middle third is the last to fuse beyond 50 years.

Second, the *coronal suture*, which is connecting the frontal bone with both parietal bones running obliquely downwards and forwards from the bregma to the pterion on either side. The coronal suture on one side (right or left) must be divided into two halves. The lower half fuses first between 40 and 50 years and the upper half fuses next between 50 and 60 years.

Third, the *lambdoid suture* which is connecting the occipital with both the parietal bones running downwards and forwards from lambda to asterion on either side, where it merges with mastooccipital and parietomastoid sutures.

The lambdoid suture on one side (right or left) must be divided into equal halves (upper and lower) by an imaginary line. The upper half fuses first between 50 and 60 years of age and the lower half fuses next between 60 and 70 years of age.

The circum-meatal sutures also completely fuse between 70 and 80 years of age.

Age Determination from Pelvis

Though the pelvic bone is more useful in sex determination age can also be established from the changes taking place sequentially from conception to the point of death.

The human pelvis is composed of right and left innominate, sacrum and coccyx to form the bony canal. Each innominate bone again is composed of three different parts. The ilium—the fan-like portion above the acetabulum, the ischium—the hard and blunt posteroinferior part that one sits on, the pubis—the anteroinferior part projecting medially to meet the opposite pubis at midline.

Each innominate bone develops from three primary and five secondary ossification centres. The ilium develops from one primary and two secondary centres, one for anteroinferior spine and another for the crest.

The pubis develops from one primary and one secondary for the ventral rami part at the symphysis.

The ischium develops from one primary and one secondary for tuberosity.

The fifth secondary ossification center (os cotyledon) is for the base of acetabulum.

The bones of the pelvis from the fetal to the adult age undergo chronological changes of age which is the basis to estimate the age during growth phase up to adulthood.

Beyond the adult age process of remodeling of bone occurs over the symphyseal part of the pubic bone that is useful in estimating the age up to 70 years.

The primary ossification centre for ilium appears at 3rd month, ischium 4th month and pubis 5th month of intrauterine period. These three components of the immature innominate bones are held together by a Y-shaped ligament called *triradiate cartilage*. The first fusion takes place between ischium and pubis at the age of 6 years whereby the ischio-pubic ramus unites.

The next phase of bone growth takes place over the triradiate cartilage which is connecting the three components. The process of ossification commences at pubertal age (13 years), and gets completed at the age of 15. By the same time between 14 and 16 years of age, the centre for anterior inferior iliac spine and centre for crest of the ilium appears. The bone formation over the crest takes place in a linear manner anteroposteriorly connecting the anterior and posterior superior iliac spines over a span of two years. After the complete formation of this epiphyseal bone, it gets fused with the body of ilium by 18 years completely.

The secondary ossification centre for ischial tuberosity also appears between 16 and 18 years of age and fusion takes place between 18 and 20 years of age. The secondary centre for pubis develops as a ventral ramp little later, i.e. after 20 years and contribute to the maturation of pubic symphysis late in life. Once the maturation process is over, morphological changes occurring over the symphyseal face are useful in age determination. These morphological changes are studied with 5 components of the pubic symphysis. They are:

1. Symphyseal face
2. Dorsal margin
3. Ventral margin
4. Superior and
5. Inferior extremities

The morphological changes affecting each component is categorised into 6 stages or phases of which first three enable to identify individuals up to 40 years and last three enable to calculate the older age group.

The first feature to be observed in the symphyseal face which is elevated with clearly marked transverse ridges separated by furrows in young individuals. As age advances the ridges and furrows gradually disappears with fine granular appearance of the symphyseal face and finally has irregular shape in advanced age.

The second component, the ventral and the dorsal margins, is absent in young individuals but everted elevation appears as limbs first over the dorsal margin and completes at the upper part of ventral margin in old age.

The third component, the upper and lower extremities, is absent in young individuals but become prominent in old age.

With these dimorphism the age can be determined from 2nd to 7th decade approximately.

Age Determination from Scapula

Age changes in the scapula can be studied under two headings
1. Ossification changes after maturity
2. Atrophic changes after maturity

Ossification Changes After Maturity

(a) Lipping of circumferential margin of glenoid cavity occurs between 30 and 35 years.
(b) Lipping of clavicular facet occurs at 35–40 years.
(c) Plaque formation on the undersurface of acromial process occurs at 40–45 years.
(d) Increasing demarcation of base of scapular spine begins at or after 50 years.
(e) Appearance of cristae scapulae after 50 years.

Atrophic Changes After Maturity

(a) Disappearance of vascular lines: Fine lines of superficial and deep vascularity distinctly visible up to 25 years after which they diminish gradually as age advances.
(b) Atrophic spots: Areas of bone atrophy either localised or discretely seen especially over the infraspinous fossa which can be seen by transillumination after 45 years.

(c) Buckling and pleating: Bone absorption and distortion due to altered vascularity gives the appearance of buckling and pleating of bone over the infraspinous fossa which can be observed on illumination usually after 40 years.

Age Determination from Long Bones after Maturity

Thin section from the shafts of long bones can be examined under low-powered microscope to study the structural changes associated with advancement of age in the outer third of the cortex for the following components.

1. Number of osteones
2. Number of fragmented osteones
3. Percentage of circumferential lamellar bone
4. Number of non-haversian canals.

The first two components increase with advancing age and the second two components decrease with advancing age and disappear completely after 55 to 60 years.

ESTIMATION OF STATURE

Stature is one of the universal characters of biological profile of an individual. Estimation of stature is much more difficult than it appears, since it is highly variable and influenced by several factors such as nutrition, heredity, environment and diseases during life and after death the physical state of the bones also changes. From birth to adulthood stature increases until a maximum is reached beyond which it decreases in old at an average rate of 0.6 mm for every one year of advancement of age due to shrinkage of bone and vertebral discs.

The most common method for estimating stature is the regression equation formula from measurement of the long limb bones. When a single bone is used to calculate, it is called simple regression equation and when several bones are used, it is called multiple regression equation. The most reliable bones to determine the height are the lower limb bones of which femur is the best.

1. Length of the bone should be measured with the help of Hepburn's osteometric board. This length is multiplied with a multiplication factor and product is added with a constant factor.
   For example, femur length $\times$ 2.11 + 70.35
   There are two formulae based on this mathematical equation analysis invented by Karl Pearson and Trotter and Gleser. These factors differ in different races, different states of bone and different types of bone.
2. Anatomical method or fully method: Skeletal height measured from skull to calcaneum individually as follows.
   Skull height (bregma to basion) (Figs 6.17 and 6.18).
   Vertebral column (C_2 to S_1)
   Femur
   Tibia
   Talus
   Calcaneum
   Sum up all and add 10.8 $\pm$ 2 for soft tissues.

To measure height of skull

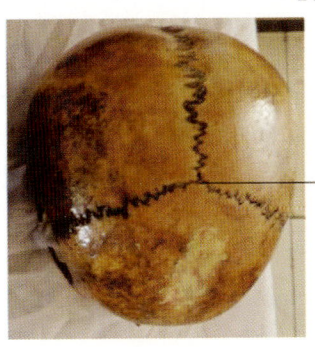

Bregma (highest point to calculate stature)

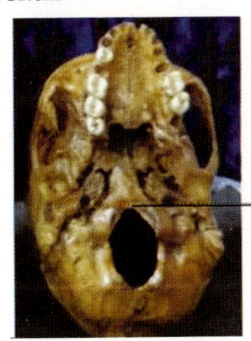

Basion (lowest point to calculate stature)

Fig. 6.17   **Fig. 6.18**

3. For Indians there are two different formulas for wet and dry bones.
   The formula based on length of a given long bone has a proportion of stature invented by Topinard and Pan. The wet bones are used and it should be measured in inches.

   Humerus   20%
   Tibia   22% } to the total height
   Fibula   22%
   Femur   27%

   Nat method is suited for dry bones, maximum length measured in inches for each bone and multiplied with a multiplication factor as follows.
   Humerus × 5.30
   Radius × 6.90
   Ulna × 6.30
   Femur × 3.70
   Tibia and fibula × 4.48

DETERMINATION OF ETHNICITY OR RACIAL AFFINITY

The race is defined as a group of population sharing common social, cultural and physical attributes.

Based on the above facts the world human population has been classified into three primary racial groups as Negroid, Caucasoid, and Mongoloid. Because of frequent migration and intermixing of population, modern anthropologist identified 5 biological groups as

1. Mongoloid (Chinese and Japanese)
2. Negroid (Africans and American Blacks)
3. Caucasoids (Europeans, West Asians and Asian Indians)
4. Australoids (Australians)
5. Polynesians (Mixed racial groups)

The morphological characters which reflect the racial traits are mostly found on the craniofacial skeleton. The shape of the head, length and breadth of the face, nasal aperture, orbits, malar prominence and mandibular morphology are more useful in racial discrimination which are tabulated in Table 6.3.

Table 6.3: Morphological characters reflecting racial traits

	Negroid	*Caucasoid*	*Mongolian*
1. Head shape	Long and narrow	Neither long nor round	Round and broad
2. Face	Anterior projection (Facial prognathism)	Flat face (orthognathism)	Mid-facial projection
3. Nasal opening	Wide	Narrow	Medium and flat
4. Nasal sill	Guttered	Sharp edged	Smooth
5. Mandible	Prominent with forward projection	Projecting chin	Receding chin
6. Orbital shape	Rectangular	Triangular	Rounded
7. Interorbital distance	Wider	Medium	Narrow
8. Cephalic index	Dolicocephalic (70–74.9)	Mesaticephalic (75–79.9)	Brachycephalic (80–85)
9. Shape of palate	Rectangular	Triangular	Horseshoe shaped
10. Bones of extremities	Distal (forearms and legs) part tends to be longer than the proximal (arms and thighs)	Shorter	Shorter
(a) Radius to humerus ratio	High	Low	Low
(b) Tibia to femur ratio	High	Low	Low
(c) Anteroposterior curvature of femur	Absent	Obvious	Not obvious

DATING OF BONES (TIME SINCE DEATH)

Introduction

Dating of bone denotes the time lapsed after death, which can be determined by physio-chemical changes that occur in the bone after death. After death all the soft tissues disappear leaving behind the bones by decomposition process. But the decomposition process continues in the bone till the bones are converted into dust and debris with striking physical changes, very slowly. These decaying changes are helpful to determine the dating of bone or time since death. These changes can be observed by the following methods.

1. Physical appearance
2. Physical test
3. Biochemical test
4. Serological test
5. Immunological test
6. DNA study

These decaying changes form the basis for determination of time lapsed after death which is more crucial for homicidal investigation to create a strong alibi against the accused/suspect.

Methods of Examination

Visual Test

Bone should be examined for the following physical characters.

1. Soft tissues remnants
2. Weight
3. Colour
4. Texture
5. Odour

1. *Soft Tissue Remnants*

Recent bones will have attached soft tissues in the form of tendons, ligaments and cartilages especially at the ends and articular surfaces. These will become dry gradually to break into dust, quickly occurs when the bones are exposed; delayed in water and much late over the buried bones.

2. *Weight*

Heaviness (weight) of the bone depends upon the collagenous stroma which undergoes gradual reduction with increasing time till complete loss whereby the bones become lighter.

3. *Colour*

Colour of a fresh bone is deep yellow, the intensity of the colour gradually becomes lighter from ends of the bone towards the shaft till the whole became white evenly.

4. *Texture*

The fresh bone feels smooth and greasy (green bone) but loss of periosteum with advancing time, the bone becomes rough and dry.

5. *Odour*

Fresh bone emits strong odour of decay and as the time passes the intensity of the odour gradually becomes less and finally becomes odourless.

All the above physical characters gradually disappear at varying periods depending upon several factors mainly the environment and the type of the bone, approximately from one year to several decades.

Physical Test

UV lamp test: Shaft of a long bone is cut across and the cut end should be examined in the dark under ultraviolet lamp. A fresh bone emits silvery blue flourescence from the cut surface. As the time increases after death this fluorescence disappears from periphery towards the centre and also outwards from around the marrow cavity. This progression of non-fluorescence gradually involves the whole thickness of the cortical bone due to gradual loss of organic stroma. This process will take approximately 100–150 years.

Biochemical Tests

1. Nitrogen

Fresh bone contains about 4.5 percent nitrogen which progressively diminishes with increasing time after death. The level of nitrogen content falls to 4 percent at the end of 100 years and 2.5 percent in 350 years and complete loss will take more than 500 years.

2. Amino Acids

The proteins present in the bone collagen can be converted into amino acids by treating with heated hydrochloric acid. Fresh bone contains about 15 amino acids and this number drops progressively as the interval after death increases. Of all the acids proline and hydroxyproline vanish within 50 years after death, whereas the acid loss takes a long time even up to centuries.

3. Serological Test

Detection of blood pigments from the bone with benzedine or phenophthalein reagents is positive only up to 100 years.

Immunological Test

Bone powder diluted with weak ammonia and vacuum concentrated, contains antigen. This antigen when treated with anti-human serum which contains the antibody, antigen–antibody reaction takes place at their junction (either by gel diffusion or electrophoresis). A positive reaction between the two fluids indicates the bone belongs to a person who died within 5–10 years only.

Radiocarbon Test

Carbon exists in two isotopic forms C_{14} and C_{12} in a ratio of $1:1$ billion. The C_{14} is radioactive and unstable, whereas the C_{12} is stable. This C_{14} enters the body through food and water from the atmosphere to maintain the ratio with C_{12} fairly constant. After death the C_{14} absorption is ceased and its level in the body gradually falls. The half-life of C_{14} is about 5700 years and after this period the C_{14} to C_{12} ratio will be $1:2000$ million. This change in the C_{14} to C_{12} ratio takes a longer duration even up to 100 thousand years which is more useful in archaeological study and is no way useful in solving medicolegal problems.

CAUSE OF DEATH

Death Due to Trauma

After ascertaining the approximate time since death one should take effort to determine the cause of death from the available bones. In order to find out violent traumatic deaths the bones are put into two categories as protective bones and supportive bones. Obviously the bones which harbor the vital organs such as brain, brain stem, larynx, lungs and heart with major blood vessels are called protective bones and bones of extremities are called supportive bones.

Evidence of trauma caused either by blunt or sharp weapon over the protective bones indicates the cause of death obviously provided it is proved as antemortem by benzidine or phenolphthalein reagent.

Injury to the supportive bones may prove fatal only when left untreated for a long time. Otherwise, it may incapacitate the victim to defend or escape and if left unattended death results from exsanguination after several hours. However, by corroborating the ante-mortem data such as last seen alive and circumstances surrounding the death and confessional statement of the accused with the findings of the bones can lead to ascertain the death cause and manner accurately.

Non-traumatic Deaths

Death due to poisoning: Death caused due to poisons mainly heavy metals especially arsenic can be detected by chemical analysis even after centuries from the bones.

Deaths in conflagration: Detection of carboxyhaemoglobin from bone marrow is possible in death due to ante-mortem burns and carbon monoxide inhalation.

Drowning deaths: Detection of diatoms from bone marrow is a proof of ante-mortem drowning.

In determination of cause of death a thorough search for signs of violence on the bones especially cranium, upper cervical vertebrae, neck skeleton, thoracic cage should be made out along with the bones of the extremities. If no signs of violence, the bones especially the long bones should be sent for toxicological analysis in accordance with the circumstances surrounding the death. For example, if the bones are partly burnt, test for carboxyhaemoglobin and if the bones are recovered from water do diatom test.

Child Abuse Deaths

Evidence of chronic child abuse can be classically seen over the skeletal remains of victims of child abuse deaths as lone or combination of the following:

1. Multiple fracture on different bones especially limb bones, ribs, etc. at varying stages of healing.
2. Harris lines: Fine markings at the growing ends of the long bones indicating temporary arrest of growth due to prolonged illness, poor nutrition and psychological stress followed by normal growth after sometime which can be detected on X-rays.

Like Harris line in long bones temporary arrest of teeth development can be seen on X-ray as fine lines called lines of Retzius.

Foetal Bones in Determination of Gestational Age

Causes of infanticide especially female infanticide are being notified or detected late after burial and on exhumation only the skeleton are often recovered. Though the criminality has to be proved only by circumstances, certain facts can be established in relation to the viability and maturity of the foetus which can also contribute valuable points for death investigation.

Viability

To determine foetal viability the following bones of the foetal skeleton must be retrieved and examined as follows.

1. Basilar part of the occipital bone: This is the excellent part of cranium to determine the viability of the foetus as the dimensions of the bone change with age of the foetus.

The anterioposterior (sagittal) length should be measured between anterior border (sphenooccipital synchondrosis) and the notch over the anterior border of foramen magnum at the back in midline (maximum length). Next the maximum breadth should be measured transversely between the lateral tubercles. The relationship between these two measurements helps in determining the viability of the foetus.

Before 7 months (non-viable), the length will be more than the breadth and after 7 months (viable), the width exceeds the length.

2. Temporal bone: The three parts of the temporal bone (squamous part, petrous part and tympanic part) develop from separate centres. The squamous and tympanic part fuses after 7 months and all the three parts fuse together at 10th month (full-term foetus).

3. Mandible: During development the mandible develops as a separate bone on each side and fuse together at the symphysis at the age of 2 years. There is a mathematical equation between the length of the mandible on one side to the total length of the foetus. The length of the mandible in millimetre is equal to the crown to heel length in centimetres. For example, if the length of mandible is 50 mm, the foetal length will be 50 cm. Thus the mandible on one side is one-tenth of the body length and by using the rule of Hasse, the age of the foetus can be ascertained.

Do all the Bones Belong to the Same Individual or Different Individuals?

To solve this problem of individualization of given bones, the inferences ascertained such as age, sex, race and stature and time since death should be compared and corroborated. If there is any discrimination in the inferences or bones of two individuals of the same age and sex died at the same time and buried in the same pit, individualization can be made out with the following methods:

1. Anatomical matching
2. Articular matching
3. UV lamp examination
4. Serological examination
5. DNA profile

With the above methods it is easy to segregate bones of different individuals but this question arises occasionally in forensic practice.

POSITIVE IDENTIFICATION

After successfully establishing the universal (biological) profile the individual (idiosyncratic) profile should be searched over the bones in order to establish the positive identity. The following antemortem data of the missing person are useful to confirm the identity of the individual positively along with the inferences of the biological features consistently.

1. Antemortem X-rays, especially the skull
2. Antemortem dental data
3. Traumatic and surgical signs on the bones
4. Occupational effects on the bones

Antemortem X-rays

Comparison of antemortem X-ray of skull with X-ray taken from the available skull can be analyzed to confirm the identity positively or to exclude. From the X-ray skull the most valuable information is complemented by frontal sinus comparison between the antemortem and post-mortem X-rays. The frontal sinus should be examined for its presence or absence (congenital), if it is present it should be assessed for size, shape and septal pattern. The frontal sinus once developed never get altered or affected by any disease during life after adulthood. The frontal sinus pattern is the best identification trait as there are no sinuses alike and that pattern is unique to that individual.

Dental Alignment

Next to the frontal sinus the dental alignment especially over the anterior teeth particularly the incisors offers best data for identity.

Antemortem Dental Data

Comparison with antemortem dental data for dental irregularities or dental imperfections or dental abnormalities or dental restorations offers valuable points to establish the positive identity. Hence, comparison of postmortem dental data with antemortem dental records such as dental X-rays and dental casts yields valuable information to fix the identity.

Frontal sinus pattern and dental data are very much helpful to fix the identification positively, hence both of them are having equal importance as the fingerprint of the individual.

Skeletal Injuries

Skeletal injuries during life whether treated or not can become a permanent marker as a deformity especially the limb bones. Surgically implants like plates or nails are also helpful to fix the identity of the individual by comparing with X-rays taken during treatment.

Occupational Evidence on Bones

Occupation also leaves some permanent alterations upon the bone. The following are the few examples of occupational evidence on bones

1. Weaver's bottom: Bony outgrowth from the ischial tuberosities due to chronic inflammation of surrounding soft tissues of weavers who are habituated to sit on hard wooden table while weaving in their looms.
2. Stenographer's bottom: Pelvis of stenographers gets wide and thicker due to prolonged typing work.
3. Florists finger tips: Arthritis affecting the finger bones of the florists
4. Milker's neck: Changes in the cervical vertebra of milkman due to shifting of cows weight while milking.
5. Electrician's tooth: Notched incisors of electrician who are used to biting and stripping of electrical cords.

The above changes in the bone can also help in the establishment of identity in a few instances.

SUPERIMPOSITION

Definition

A high-tech photography which compares a photograph of the missing person with a skull believed to belong to the missing person in the photo.

Procedure

Superimposition is done by using two video cameras connected with a mixture that can move the images on and off screen. The skull is positioned as the face in the photo with one video camera focused on the skull and the second on the photo. The mixture is connected to a TV monitor so that the images of skull and photo can be moved over one another vertically or horizontally to fix both the images into a single one.

By equalizing the fades of both the images, one can examine and compare certain points to ascertain whether the skull belongs to the person in the given photo or not. Simply it is the negatives of photo and skull that are imposed upon each other with the help of video to look for alignment of certain points on skull with the photo. For example, centre of the mandible must align with chin in the photo; the bite of teeth must align with lip line on the photo. Like that the nasal opening, orbit, auditory meatus, etc.

Medicolegal Importance

It is a semi-scientific investigation to establish the identity of a missing person from the skull. Negative inference is more valuable than the positive report because positive is only a probability, whereas negative is a conclusion.

7

Foetal Autopsy

INTRODUCTION

The union of sperm with ovum is known as fertilisation, which usually occurs in the fallopian tube. The fertilized ovum gradually moves through the fallopian tube towards uterine cavity to get implanted. This process of migration and implantation usually takes place between 7 and 10 days after fertilization. Implantation that occurs anywhere other than the uterine cavity results in ectopic pregnancy.

The fertilised ovum grows in the uterus after gaining attachment into the endometrium by finger-shaped outgrowths called chorionic villi. If the process of this attachment is interfered with by any inborn intrinsic or extrinsic factors, then the fertilized ovum is expelled outside. This is the reason that a pregnancy can be positively and safely declared only 7–10 days after a missed period.

Shortly after implantation, the fertilized ovum begins to grow gradually. At the third month the embryo grows into a foetus with development of placenta and the umbilical cord. The placenta provides oxygen and nourishment to the developing foetus and also carries away the foetal wastes through the umbilical cord. The embryo is enclosed by a sac of fluid called amniotic fluid which protects the growing foetus from jolts and pressure. The embryo has three germinal layers—the outer ectoderm, middle mesoderm and inner endoderm. The outer layer gives rise to the skin, brain, spinal cord and nerves. The muscles, blood vessels, heart, bones and gonadal organs arise from the middle layer and the organs of the gastro-intestinal, respiratory and urinary tracts develop from endoderm. The heart begins to beat from the 4th to 5th week of pregnancy but at this period it is impossible to hear the heart sounds. The embryo gradually increases from the size of a peanut to a fully matured foetus throughout the period of gestation. Thus the growth and development is useful to assess the age of the foetus where growth implies increase in size, while development implies gradual attainment of functional maturity. Thus the structural and functional growth goes together gradually with the advancing pregnancy in a regular sequence.

WHEN AND WHY A DEAD FOETUS HAS TO BE EXAMINED?

Whenever a dead foetus either fresh or decomposed is found abandoned or discarded, it is the challenging duty of the medical officer to ascertain the following points by a meticulous examination.

- First the gestational age has to be assessed
- Second whether the foetus attained viability or not
- Third whether the foetus was born alive or dead (in case of viable foetus)
- Fourth period of survival ⎫
- Fifth the cause of death ⎭ (if born alive)

After ascertaining all the above points, a reasonable guidance can be extended to police to trace the biological mother.

In cases of unwanted pregnancy leading to childbirth when it occurs unmarried girls, widows or sometimes in divorced women, the foetus used to be discarded or abandoned. If the pregnancy is detected beyond the maximum period of Medical Termination of Pregnancy (MTP), or after an unsuccessful abortion, delivery may sometimes be conducted far away from their residence and the foetus is then killed and discarded.

A discarded foetus attracts the attention of passer by or some domestic animals which may drag out or even destroy the body. However, when the dead foetus is seized by police, further investigations can be carried out only after a foetal autopsy. The doctor who performs the autopsy should opine about the age, sex, state of viability, whether born dead or alive in case of viable foetus and the cause of death with the period of survival also in case of live born. Hence the knowledge of development and foetal maturation is essential to ascertain all the above mentioned factors.

ASSESSMENT OF AGE FROM FOETAL GROWTH

The age of the foetus can be ascertained by various body measurements such as crown-heel length (CHL), crown-rump length, head circumference, chest circumference and foot length. In foetal autopsy the age of the foetus is usually estimated by measuring the length, from crown to heel in centimetres with stretched knee joint. From this crown-heel length, the age of the foetus is calculated according to Rule of Hasse where the length of the foetus is less than 25 cm, the square root of the length is the age of the foetus in lunar months.

For example, crown-heel length is 9 cm, age of the foetus is $\sqrt{9}$ = 3 months

Crown-heel length is 16 cm, age of the foetus is $\sqrt{16}$ = 4 months

Crown-heel length is 25 cm, age of the foetus is $\sqrt{25}$ = 5 months

If the crown-heel length is 23 cm, the square root crossed is 4 (16 cm) and the next square root is 5 (25 cm). Hence the age is above 4 months and below 5 months.

When the length is more than 25 cm, one-fifth of the length is the age of the foetus in months.

For example, the length of the foetus: 35 cm
Age of the foetus: 7 months

If the crown-heel length is 38 cm, the age is above 7 months and below 8 months.

If the length is measured in inches, then twice the crown-heel length gives the age of the foetus in weeks. For example, CHL = 9 inches × 2 = 18 weeks.

After ascertaining the approximate age from the growth, this should be confirmed with the developmental changes which also vary in accordance with the advancing gestational period, representing the process of maturation from the day of conception till delivery.

Figures 7.1 to 7.10 are helpful to illustrate the developmental changes beginning from the first month to the 10th month of gestation.

First Month (Fig. 7.1)

- The length of the embryo is 1 cm.
- The eyes are seen as two dark spots.
- The mouth is seen as a cleft.
- The arms and legs are seen as tiny buds (limb buds).

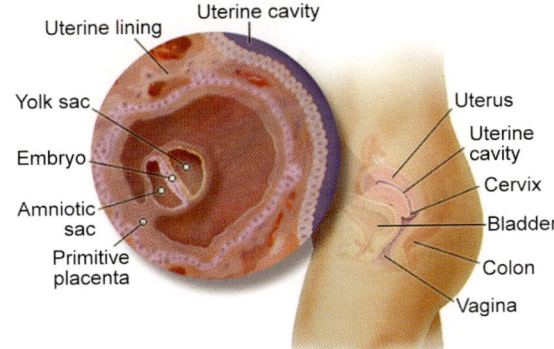

Fig. 7.1: First month of gestation

Second Month (Fig. 7.2)

- The length is 4 cm.
- The anus is seen as a dark spot at the caudal end.
- Webbed fingers and toes are seen on the hands and feet.

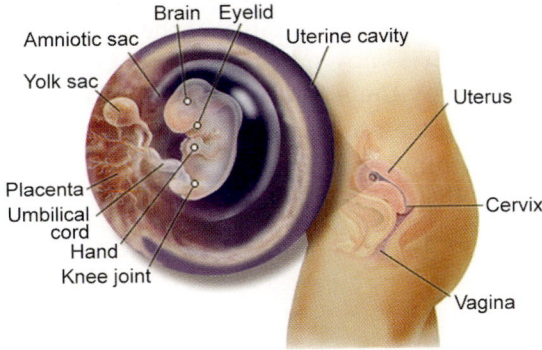

Fig. 7.2: Second month of gestation

Third Month (Fig. 7.3)

- The crown-heel length is 9 cm.
- Facial features become distinctly human.
- The head and trunk are demarcated by a distinct neck.
- The fingers and toes are more distinct with soft membranous nails.
- Eyes are distinct with eyelids and covered by papillary membrane.

- The umbilical cord and placental are fully formed.
- **External genitalia:** Bisexual character present, hence sex cannot be determined.
- **Medicolegal importance:** According to MTP Act 1975 up to 12 weeks pregnancy can be terminated by a registered medical practitioner on valid causes.

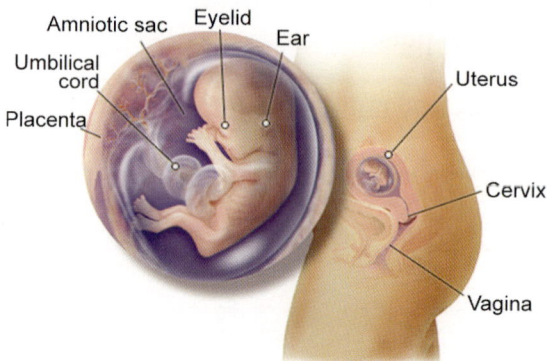

Fig. 7.3: Third month of gestation

Fourth Month (Fig. 7.4)

- The length of the foetus is 16 cm.
- Ear lobes become distinct.
- Eyebrows and eyelashes appear.
- Soft, non-pigmented fine hairs appear over the skin (lanugo hair).
- Finger creases appears.
- External genitalia are fully developed, hence sex of the foetus can now be determined.
- At this stage, as the limbs are fully developed the foetus moves and the pregnant mother can feel these movements as a *flutter*. The ability of the mother to feel the foetal movement for the first time after conception is known as quickening. **Quickening is helpful to calculate the expected date of delivery by the attending obstetrician**.
- The foetus starts swallowing the amniotic fluid and excretes it as urine.
- **Medicolegal importance:** Criminal abortion after quickening invites enhanced punishment of 7 years under Section 312 IPC.

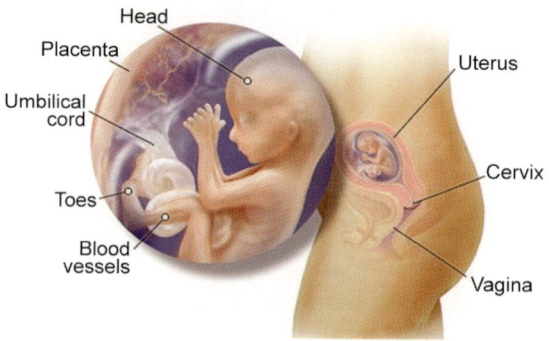

Fig. 7.4: Fourth month of gestation

Fifth Month (Fig. 7.5)

- As the growth is tremendous the crown-heel length increases from 16 cm at the end of fourth month to 25 cm at the end of fifth month.
- Scalp hair begins to appear.
- Finger nails grown well.
- Ossification centres for manubrium and 1st segment of mesosternum appear.
- Meconium is present in the bowels.
- **Medicolegal importance:** According to MTP Act 1975, 20th week is the maximum period by which the pregnancy can be terminated by two registered medical practitioners (one of whom should be a postgraduate in obstetrics and gynaecology) under valid reasons.

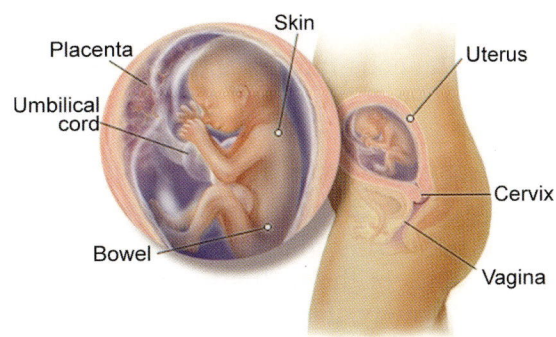

Fig. 7.5: Fifth month of gestation

Sixth Month (Fig. 7.6)

- The crown-heel length is 30 cm.
- Skin is red and wrinkled due to incomplete fat deposition under the skin.
- Vernix caseosa — a white cheese-like material covers the skin (a combination of sloughed skin with secretion of sebaceous glands).
- Toe nails grown up to the tip of toe.
- The centre for calcaneum usually appears.
- **Medicolegal importance:** Due to the advancement of neonatal care units, a foetus born after 6 months can also survive, hence the foetus becomes medically viable, however, legally not viable.

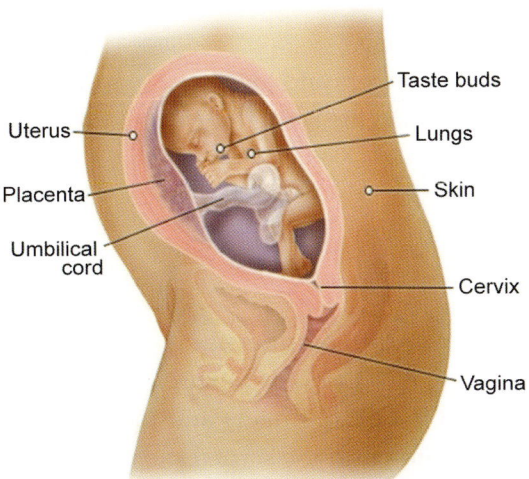

Fig. 7.6: Sixth month of gestation

Seventh Month (Fig. 7.7)

- Crown-heel length is 35 cm.
- Lanugo hair disappears from the face.
- Pupillary membrane disappears and eyelids are opened.
- Subcutaneous fat deposition is almost complete, hence the skin becomes smooth and plum.
- The finger and toe nails are thickened.
- Ossification centre for talus appears.
- Foetus attains viability (it is the physical capability of the foetus to thrive outside the uterine cavity, if born alive.) This is the period of legal viability and if born chances of survival is better and this is termed *premature birth*.

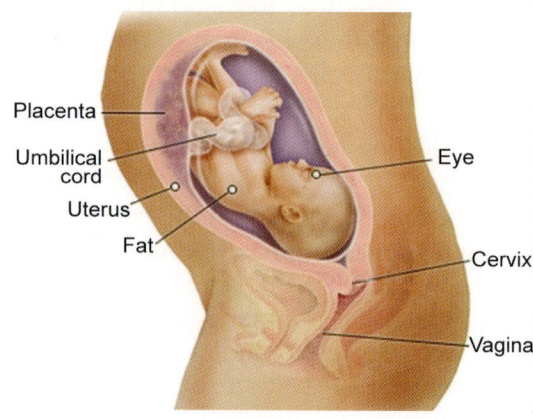

Fig. 7.7: Seventh month of gestation

- Medicolegal importance:
  1. Voluntarily causing death of a viable foetus amounts to homicide.
  2. **Stillbirth:** A baby born after viability but before full term and does not exhibit any sign of life after complete expulsion is said to be *stillborn*. All stillbirths should be registered under Registration of Birth and Death Act 1969.
  3. Ossification test for viability: Presence of ossification centres for calcaneum and talus is the proof of viability.

Eighth Month (Fig. 7.8)

- Crown-heel length is 40 cm.
- Lanugo hair begins to disappear from the parts of the body.
- Scalp hair becomes thick and coarse.
- Thick nails grow up to the tip of fingers and toes.
- In male the left testicle descends to the scrotal sac.
- The head is usually turned down.

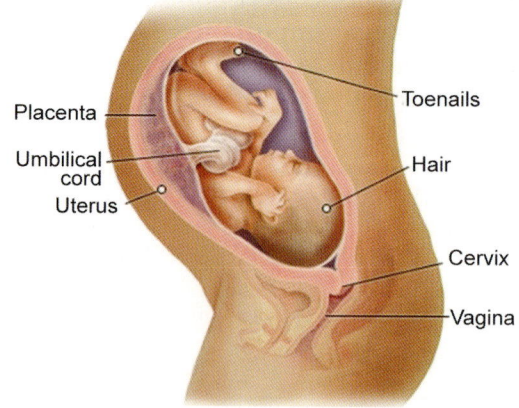

Fig. 7.8: Eighth month of gestation

Ninth Month (Fig. 7.9)

- Crown-heel length is 45 cm.
- Lanugo hair is present only over the shoulders.
- Vernix caseosa is present only over the joint flexures.
- Thick nails are grown beyond the tip of fingers and toes.
- In male the right testicle descends into the scrotal sac.
- Ossification centre for lower end of femur appears.

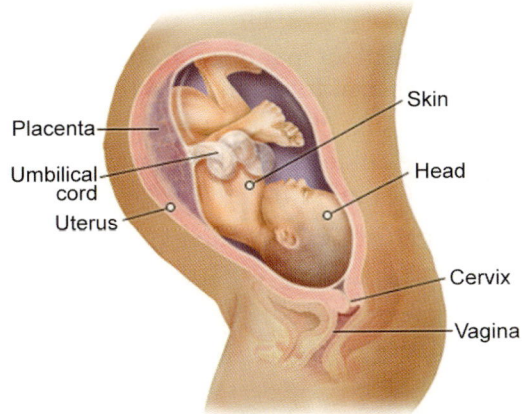

Fig. 7.9: Ninth month of gestation

Tenth Month (Fig. 7.10)

- Crown-heel length is 50 cm.
- Nails grown beyond the tip of fingers.
- Scalp hair becomes thick and coarse, grow up to 5 cm in length.
- Ossification centre for upper end of tibia appears.

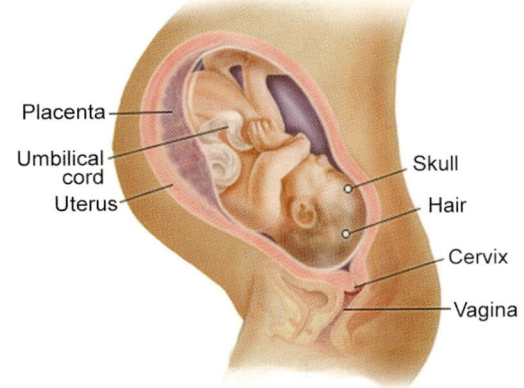

Fig. 7.10: Tenth month of gestation

The physical capability of the foetus to lead a separate existence after complete expulsion from the mother's womb is called *viability*. Though the foetus becomes viable at six months (medical viability), it must be observed under intensive medical (neonatal) care. Legally a foetus is considered as viable only after 28 weeks of pregnancy (legal viability). So, viability reflects the potential ability of the foetus to survive after birth. If the gestational age is above 7 months, then it has to be ascertained whether the child was born alive or dead.

SIGNS OF VIABILITY

The following external findings and certain ossification centres which are helpful to ascertain the viability.

1. The crown-heel length is 35 cm.
2. Scalp hair becomes thick and black.
3. Eyelids are open and pupillary membrane disappears.
4. Vernix caseosa covers the body.
5. Nails grown but not to the tip of fingers and toes.
6. Eyebrows and eyelashes are grown.

Ossification Centres

Sternum: Ossification centres are present for manubrium and the four segments of mesosternum. A vertical cut over the sternum in the middle will show the centres of ossification.

Ankle joint: A vertical cut over the sole of foot extending from the web space between 3rd and 4th toe to the heel and up to the ankle joint with a surgical knife will expose the centre for talus (7th month) and calcaneum (6th month).

Next is to assess whether the foetus was born alive or stillborn or dead born.

Live birth is the complete expulsion or extraction of a product of conception, from the uterus irrespective of the duration of pregnancy, which after such expulsion or extraction, breathes or shows any other evidence of life.

Signs of Live Birth (Autopsy Findings)

External Signs

(Probable)
1. Crown-heel length is more than 35 cm
2. Absence of pupillary membrane
3. Absence of vernix caseosa
4. Barrel-shaped chest, circumference of chest is greater than the abdomen.
5. Presence of caput succedaneum
6. Ligated umbilical cord

Internal Signs

Proof of respiration:
1. Dome of diaphragm found at the level of 7th rib.
2. Lung morphology
   (a) Pinkish in colour
   (b) Fully expanded to fill the thoracic cavities and overlying the heart except over bare area.
   (c) Soft in consistency
   (d) Rounded margins
   (e) Crepitate on palpation
   (f) Float in water (not applicable if putrefied)

Proof of deglutition:
1. Detection of air in the stomach ⎫
2. Detection of air in the duodenum ⎬ not applicable if putrefied
3. Detection of milk in the stomach and duodenum (absolute proof of live birth)
4. Detection of air in the middle ear

Proof of independent circulation:
1. Obliterated ductus arteriosus
2. Closure of foramen ovale

Signs of Live Birth during Labour

1. Cry—air passing across the vocal cord
2. Movement of limbs
3. Chest and abdominal movement due to breathing
4. Winking of eyelids
5. Apical impulse of the heart
6. Pulsation over radial, cubital, carotid, pretemporal, femoral, popliteal, anterior and posterior tibial, dorsalis pedis arteries and umbilical cord.

PROOF OF LIVE BIRTH AND SUBSEQUENT SURVIVAL BY AUTOPSY

1. Hydrostatic test (floatation test or Raygat's test): This is Breslau's first life test, the basis of which is to determine whether the lungs have respired or not by putting the whole and parts of lung into water. If they float freely, it indicates that the foetus has respired and if they sink into water, it indicates that the foetus has not respired. This test is not applicable in the decomposed (putrified) foetus.
2. Air in the stomach and also in intestine can be demonstrated by cutting them independently after tying them carefully at both ends and putting them in water bowl to see whether it floats or sink. If the foetus breathes, it also swallows air by gulping. Presence of air in the intestine is more valuable since the air is further moved into the intestine across pylorus. The air in the stomach and intestine can also be demonstrated by puncturing with a needle under water so that air escapes as bubbles. This test is also not applicable in decomposed (putrified) foetus. Then the stomach must be opened to find out the milk which is the surest sign of live birth. This is Breslau's second life test.
3. Umbilical cord: If the cord is severed close to the foetus and tied or clamped, it is a sign of live birth. The change that occurs at the stump (ring of inflammation)—dry and shriveling umbilicus indicates survival up to 5 days and umbilical stump falls after that period and complete healing occurs within 7–10 days.
4. Absence of vernix caseosa.
5. Yellowish discolouration of skin and sclera due to physiological jaundice indicates that the foetus survived more than 2 days after birth.
6. Resolving caput succedaneum. The oedematous scalp tissues over the presenting part completely resolves within 7–10 days after birth.

Internal Signs of Survival After Birth

1. Absence of meconium
2. Disappearance of nucleated red cells in the blood.
3. Falling foetal haemoglobin level
4. Circulatory changes: Closure of ductus arteriosus and foramen ovale.

Medicolegal Importance of Live Birth

1. Before declaring that a child is stillborn or dead born, resuscitation should be adequately performed since there is a possibility of physiological suspended animation.

2. In India the law presumes that every newborn found dead was born dead until the contrary is otherwise proved, and the burden of proving that the child was born alive falls on the prosecution.

3. Before framing the charge of infanticide, it should be proved that the child was born alive.

As per Barcroft statement "Breathing is living". The onset of respiration is the beginning of life after complete expulsion.

Once the fact of live birth and separate existence is proved, then the cause of death must be established by an extensive postmortem.

The foetal death may have been caused by an act of omission or an act of commission the signs of which are obviously detected by a meticulous postmortem.

Finally, the evidences which are useful to identify the biological mother must be retrieved. Mainly, the blood from umbilical vein, umbilical artery for grouping, DNA profile and mitochondrial DNA to compare with the blood of suspected mother who shows signs of recent delivery.

Stillbirth is defined as "A child born after 28 weeks of pregnancy which did not, at any time after being completely expelled from its mother, breath or show any other signs of life."

A foetus which was expelled after its death within the uterine cavity irrespective of gestational period is known as *dead born foetus*. The dead born foetus usually shows evidence of aseptic autolysis, i.e. slippage of epidermis, extreme mobility of joints, overriding of skull bones (Spalding's sign).

Once the foetus is ascertained as viable the next question is to find out whether the child is born stillborn or dead born or live born.

STILLBORN, DEAD BORN

A dead born child is one which has died in the uterus well before the delivery, irrespective of period of gestation.

Signs of Intrauterine Death

1. **Rigor mortis:** If the child shows rigor mortis after complete expulsion, it indicates that the foetus attained viability and also the death has occurred inside the uterine cavity 2–3 hours before complete expulsion.

2. **Maceration:** The term maceration denotes aseptic breakdown of foetal tissues that has occurred after the foetal death within the uterine cavity but the foetus being expelled 2–3 days after death. The earliest signs of IUD are skin slippage and dark discolouration of the umbilical cord that occurs usually within a few hours after death of the foetus in uterine cavity. If the mother's abdomen is X-rayed, gas bubbles can be seen in the great vessels (IVC, aorta, etc.) of the foetus which is also an earliest sign. Maceration is the surest sign of intrauterine death. If the foetus remains inside the uterus after death for more than a day, then this process of aseptic autolysis affect the foetal tissues to gives rise the signs of maceration. If the dead foetus is expelled within 24 hours after its death, no sign of maceration will be present.

Difference between stillborn and dead born: The essential difference between dead born and stillborn is that death of the foetus occurs inside the uterus irrespective of gestational age in the former, whereas in the later the death of the foetus occurs outside the uterine cavity (i.e. in the birth canal) during the process of normal parturition only after viability. Both the condition shows no air in the lung. There will be no sign of maceration in stillborn since it is not within the uterine cavity and not surrounded by liquor amni as in the case of dead born.

Signs of Maceration

1. Discolouration of umbilical cord (purplish black from the normal whitish yellow).
2. Skin slippage on digital pressure. Brownish red or bluish red in colour with a few blebs may also be present.
3. Body becomes soft and flaccid emitting a sweetish disagreeable odour.
4. Muscles become soft and pinkish.
5. The joints are extremely mobile and soft tissue attached around the bones will be easily separable.
6. Spalding's sign: The sutures in the vault of the cranium becomes loose and override each other which will be visualised with X-ray of mother's abdomen. This important radiological sign of skull bones realigning and overlapping is known as Spalding's sign.
7. Brain becomes pulpy and pinkish red in colour.
8. All the internal organs become flaccid with reddish purple fluid collection in the serous cavities.

EVALUATORY QUESTIONS

1. **What is infanticide?**

   Deliberate killing of a child below one year of age is known as infanticide.

2. **What is foeticide?**

   Deliberate killing of a foetus before it is born alive/deliberate killing of a foetus in utero.

3. **What is filicide?**

   Killing of a child by its own parents is known as filicide.

4. **What is neonaticide?**

   Killing a child which is born alive within a month after birth is neonaticide.

5. **What is quickening?**

   First perception of foetal movements by the pregnant women usually occurring at 16th week of pregnancy is known as quickening.

   MLI: Enhanced punishment in case of criminal abortion up to 7 years imprisonment under Section 312 IPC.

6. **What is viability?**

   Physical capability of the foetus to lead an independent life after complete expulsion from the uterus is known as viability; usually it occurs after 28th week or 7 lunar months of pregnancy.

   MLI: Causing death of a viable child is amounting to culpable homicide punishable with imprisonment up to 10 years under Section 316 IPC.

7. **What is superfecundation?**

   Superfecundation is the fertilization of two ova of the same cycle but by sperms of two different persons.

   MLI: It is a proof of adultery.

8. **What is atavism?**

   The features of the child do not resemble its immediate parents but resembling its grandparents is known as atavism.

9. **What is superfoetation?**

   Pregnancy occurs in a woman who is already pregnant.

10. **What is pseudocyesis?**

    A woman who is presumed herself to be pregnant but not so really.

Toxicology

Section

3

8

Preservation of Viscera

INTRODUCTION

Poisoning is one of the most frequent medical emergencies and a major cause of death. As we are living in constant threat of poisons of nature and manmade, it is mandatory to identify the poisons that enters into human body by collecting appropriate body fluids (excretions and secretions) in the living, and body tissues and organs from the dead.

It is the important duty of a physician in emergency department to be wise and cautious in handling a case of poisoning. Though the dictum of "Treat the patient not the poison" is to be followed, identification of poison is also most essential to interpret with the clinical manifestations and also to administer appropriate antidote. Likewise preservation of visceral organs and other body fluids is equally important to identify and quantify the poison that causes death or contribute to death and also to answer the legal queries related to death. Hence a basic knowledge about poisons is most essential in solving the medical and legal problems related to illness and death due to poisons.

What is a Poison?

A poison is defined as any substance which gains entry into human body by any means and causing illness, injury or death by its deleterious effect.

How are the Poisons Classified?

Poisons are classified easily based on their major site and type of action as follows.

1. Corrosives
   - Acid: H_2SO_4, HCl, HNO_3, carbolic acid, oxalic acid
   - Alkali: NaOH, KOH, NH_4OH,

2. Irritants
   - Organic
     - Plant: Castor, calotropis, abrus, crotin, jatropa, semicarpus
     - Animal: Snake, scorpion, bees, spider, wasps, millipede.
   - Inorganic
     - Metallic: Arsenic, lead, mercury, copper, zinc, etc.
     - Non-metallic: Phosphorous
   - Mechanical: Glass powder, diamond dust and chopped hair

3. Neurotics:

   A. Cerebral
   - Somniferous (opium, morphine, heroin, pethidine, fortwin)
   - Inebrient (ethyl alcohol, methyl alcohol, cannabis, chloral hydrate)
   - Delirient (datura)
   - Excitator (cocaine, amphetamine)

   B. Spinal: Strychnine

   C. Peripheral: Conium, curare

4. Cardiac: Aconite, oleander, digitalis, nicotine, quinine, cyanides
5. Asphyxiants: Carbon monoxide, carbon dioxide, hydrogen sulphide, methane, indane and war gases.
6. Gastrointestinal: Food poisoning
7. Hepatotoxic: Phosphorous, carbon tetrachloride
8. Nephrotoxic: Cantharides, mercury, oxalates
9. Drugs: Analgesics (paracetamol, salicylates), antibiotics, anti-depressants (imipremaine, lithium), anxiolytics (alprazolam)
10. Insecticides: Organophosphorous, carbamate, pyrethroids, etc.

ROUTE OF ENTRY, MECHANISM OF ACTION

Poisons gain entry into the body by several ways:
1. Ingestion (GI tract—solid and liquid forms)
2. Inhalation (respiratory tract—volatile poisons, dust and smoke)
3. Inoculation—introduction into the natural orifices of the body other than nose and mouth (rectum, vagina and urethra)
4. Inunctions (intact skin): For example, phenol, OPC
5. Injection (liquid poisons): Intradermal, subcutaneous, intramuscular, intravenous, intra arterial, intrathecal.

Mechanism of Action of Poisons

1. Local action: Toxic effect only at the site of contact, e.g. sulphuric acid, glass powder.
2. Systemic action: No effect at the site of contact but deleterious effect only after absorption into the system, e.g. opium, alcohol, cyanide
3. Combined effect: Toxic effect both at the site of contact and after absorption into the system, e.g. arsenic, carbolic acid, oxalic acid, phosphorous.

DUTIES OF A DOCTOR IN POISONING CASES

Medical Duties

1. Accept the patient immediately, since it is a medical emergency.
2. Assessment of general, and vital parameters (to inform the relatives about the condition)
3. No guarantee or false hope shall be given.
4. Do not withhold diagnosis and treatment for want of money.
5. Act swiftly to stabilize the patient by ABCD maneuver along with symptomatic management.

6. Administer appropriate antidotes if the poison is known.
7. Once the crisis is over, either consult or transfer the patient for further management under the care of a physician.
8. Arrange for psychiatric counselling before discharging the patient with an advice of periodical evaluation.
9. If there is no adequate facilities, administer first aid in preventing further exposure to poison and to stabilise the vital parameters and then transfer the patient with proper referral letter for further institutional management.

Legal Duties

1. Make an entry in the accident register.
2. Intimate to the police (mandatory in homicidal poisonings).
3. Preserve the first sample of stomach wash fluid.
4. Preserve the vomitus, blood and urine for analytical purpose.
5. Record dying declaration in homicidal poisoning.
6. In the event of death, body should not be handed over to the relatives.
7. No death certificate should be issued.
8. Death intimation to be given immediately to the police.
9. All the materials retrieved from the patient should be handed over to the police after getting due acknowledgement.
10. Copy of the case sheet along with the accident register should be given for further investigation.

Autopsy Protocol in Poisoning Death

1. Written authorisation from competent authority.
2. Soiled clothings, drained stains of body fluids should be properly collected and preserved for analytical purposes.
3. Examine the dead body from head to toe to rule out the possibility of forcible feeding of poison and also to rule out general and genital violence.
4. It is mandatory to select, collect and preserve the appropriate visceral organs and body fluids such as blood, urine, and vitreous for chemical analysis during autopsy.

INDICATIONS FOR VISCERA PRESERVATION

1. Proved cases of death due to poison (clinically established) or confirmed circumstantially.
2. Suspected poisoning death
3. All cases of sudden natural death
4. All homicidal death
5. All suspicious death
6. Death occurring at workplace
7. Death due to RTA where death occurs within 24 hours after the accident
8. Death due to animal bite or sting
9. Exhumation
10. Custodial death

11. Death which entitled monetary compensation
12. In cases of all unknown deaths
13. Deaths in which no obvious cause can be determined (obscure or unwitnessed deaths)
14. Death due to criminal abortion.

Purpose of Viscera Preservation

1. To identify the poison.
2. Whether the poison has caused the death or it has contributed to the death (causative factor or contributive factor)
3. To exclude poison in cases of death without obvious causes.
4. To rule out poison in cases of sudden natural death
5. To rule out poison in homicidal cases (conclusion by process of exclusion)

Selection of Tissues and Organs

To avoid unwanted organ retrieval for detection of poison, basic information regarding the type of poison is necessary. If the type and nature of the poison is not known, circumstances surrounding the death can help to search and select the organ to be retrieved.

However, the objective evidences observed during meticulous postmortem examination is more important in order to corroborate with history, circumstances and analytical aspect. Wrongful selection of body tissues and faulty preservation will seriously hamper the opinion regarding the cause, mode and manner of death which ultimately leads to miscarriage of justice. Hence knowledge of viscera preservation is essential for the doctors who are handling medicolegal autopsies.

Selection of organs is mainly based on the route of entry of poison and physiological role of organs, which helps in propulsion of poisons to undergo bio-conversion or bio-transmission till elimination.

Site of Reception

The ingested poison is carried to stomach through the oesophagus. The role of stomach in most of the ingested poison is only to receive and allow the poison to stay for sometime which may extend from a few minute to a few hours depends upon physical state of poison and condition of the stomach. Stomach is not the site of absorption for most of the poisons except a few such as cyanide, nicotine sulphate and alcohol to a lesser extent. Because of the above facts as long as the poison stays in the stomach it has to be considered as outside the body. Elimination of poison which will save the patient from deleterious effect of poisoning which can be done either by inducing emesis or evacuation by gastric lavage. If the poison is not removed from stomach, it will be emptied into the duodenum through the pyloric sphincter which is controlled by neural and hormonal reflexes only during life, not after death certainly.

RETRIEVAL OF STOMACH

Stomach should be mobilized gently from its attachments and omentum. Apply two ligature 1 cm away from each over the cardiac end (above the gastroesophageal junction) and another such ligature over the pyloric end (gastroduodenal junction) of the stomach with thick thread and then cut in between the ligatures at both the sites and remove the stomach to a clean plastic or enamel tray (Fig. 8.1). This procedure of stomach removal ensures no spillage or loss of stomach contents.

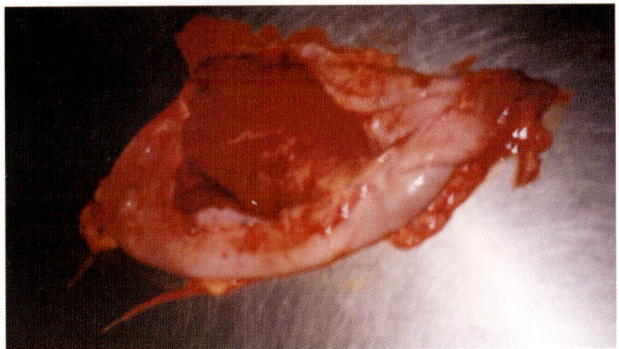

Fig. 8.1: Retrieval of stomach

Next step is to open the stomach along the greater curvature from cardiac to pyloric end and empty the contents into a tray. Examine the quantity, colour and odour and state of digestion if food particles are present. Examine the gastric mucosa to know whether it is congested or hyperemic, eroded, echymotic, haemorrhagic and search for remnants of poison in-between the mucosal folds. All the above findings must be documented carefully. In adults, half of the contents with half of the stomach and in children, whole stomach and its contents should be preserved.

Points to Remember

1. Detection of poison in the stomach is a mere proof of consumption.
2. If the victim survived long and/or treated subsequent to the consumption, no poison will be present in the stomach.
3. Detection of poison in the stomach during autopsy indicates either the patient died before the medical treatment or gastric lavage has not been performed in spite of survival under treatment in the hospital which amounts to criminal negligence.
4. Prognosis in poisoning cases depends upon the shortest interval between consumption and medical intervention (golden hours).
5. It is not uncommon that poison may be introduced into the stomach to mislead investigation in homicidal deaths. Hence detection of poison in the stomach alone is not a proof of poison consumed by the victim, which may be administered after the victim was killed by some other means without having any external signs of violence.

Site of Absorption—Small Intestine

The poison which enters into the intestine is gradually absorbed into the portal venous system because the small intestine is the site of absorption.

The upper end of the small intestine not less than 100 cm should be collected after ligating both the ends to prevent the spillage or loss of contents (Fig. 8.2). After putting into the tray the intestine must be opened along the antimesentric border and the contents must be examined for quantity, colour and odour. The mucosa must also be examined for any evidence of erosion inflammation and perforation and then transfer it to a wide mouthed clean dry glass jar. Preservative should be added.

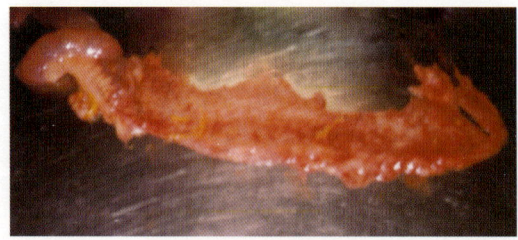

Fig. 8.2: Intestine

Points to be Remembered

1. Detection of poison in the intestine is a proof of survival of the victim after consumption of poison.
2. Mere detection of poison in the intestine is not an absolute proof of death due to poison.
3. The intestine should be preserved in a separate container in order to differentiate whether the poison was consumed before death or introduced after death by the criminal to mislead the investigation.
4. The poisons which cause death quickly such as cyanide, nicotine sulphate may not be detected in the intestine.
5. No poison can be detected in the intestine in cases of injected poisons, and poisons inoculated through rectum or vagina except for opium and opioids (enterohepatic circulation).

Site of Detoxication

The absorbed poison from the intestine is carried by the portal veins to the liver. In the liver, poison undergoes detoxication by various biochemical processes. 80% of the absorbed poison after detoxification in the liver along with the undetoxicated poison enters into the systemic circulation through the hepatic system. Hence the liver is the site of detoxification of poisons

RETRIEVAL OF LIVER

Liver tissue not less than 300–500 gm comprising both right and left lobe should be retrieved and collected in a wide mouthed clean glass jar after making it into small pieces (Fig. 8.3).

Points To Remember

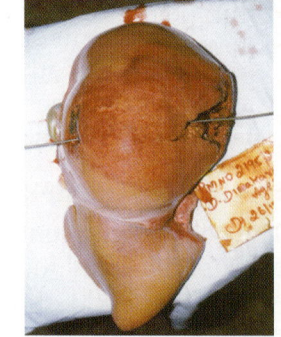

1. Detection of poison in the liver is also a proof of poisoning and survival after consumption at least for a few hours irrespective of the route of entry.
2. Poison may not be detected if the victim survived for a long time after consumption and also in treated cases.
3. Detection of poison in the liver is a proof that poison may cause the death or hastens the death.

Fig. 8.3: Retrieval of liver

Site of Excretion

The poison both detoxicated and un-detoxicated enters the systemic circulation through hepatic veins and gets evenly distributed to all parts of the body and finally gets excreted mainly through the kidney which is the main portal of excretion irrespective of nature and route of entry of poison.

RETRIEVAL OF KIDNEY

The kidneys are retrieved properly without any adherent fat tissues (Fig. 8.4). Longitudinal half of each kidney in adults and both kidneys in children must be retrieved. Retrieved kidney can be put together with liver in the same container.

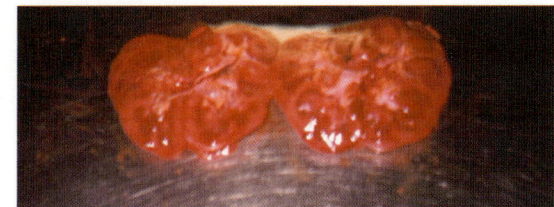

Fig. 8.4: Retrieval of kidney

Points to Remember

1. Detection of poison in kidney is an absolute proof of poisoning irrespective of route of administration and survival after its administration.
2. To avoid the possibility of non-functioning of any one of the kidneys, halves of both kidneys should be preserved in adults.

   In cases of ingested poisons the above said organs should be collected routinely irrespective of the type of poison ingested.

SPECIAL ORGANS TO BE COLLECTED

Apart from the above said routine organs, certain other special organs must also be collected according to the type of poison ingested:

Brain

One-half of the brain including cerebellum, midbrain, and pons should be collected in all cases of death due to the following neurotoxic poisons (Fig. 8.5):

- Carbolic acid
- Morphine, pethidine, heroin
- Barbiturate, alcohols
- Organophosphorous compounds
- Anesthetic agents
- Suspected drug abuse deaths
- Cyanide poisoning

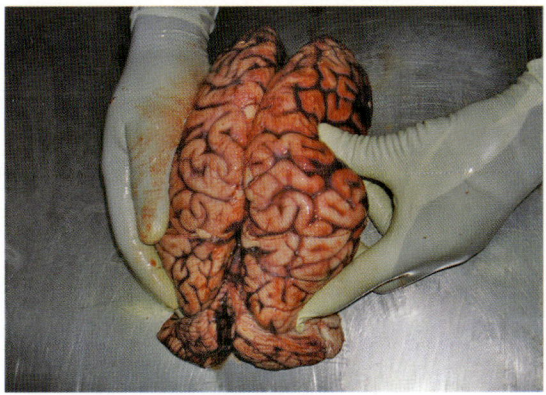

Fig. 8.5: Brain

Spinal Cord

Retrieve the spinal cord by anterior or posterior approach in cases of death due to strychnine and gelsemium poisoning.

Heart

Right half of the heart or the whole heart can be preserved in cases of death due to cardiac poisons such as aconite, oleander, etc. (Fig. 8.6).

Fig. 8.6: Heart

Muscles

The ideal site to retrieve sufficient muscle mass is the gluteal region. In case of death due to OPC, or muscle relaxants (succinyl choline), the gluteal muscle may be preserved for detection especially in decomposed bodies.

Hair, Nails and Bone (Fig. 8.7)

Since heavy metal poisons, especially arsenic and thallium, get deposited in hair, nail, and keratin tissues, which should be retrieved in all cases of death due to heavy metal poisoning both in acute and chronic cases.

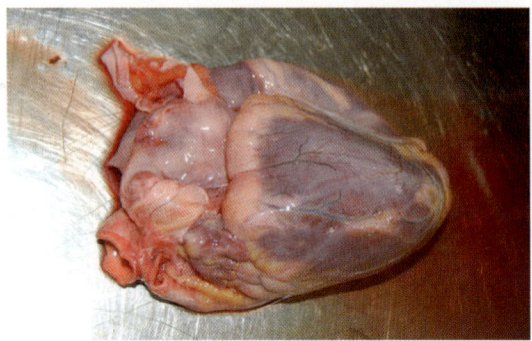

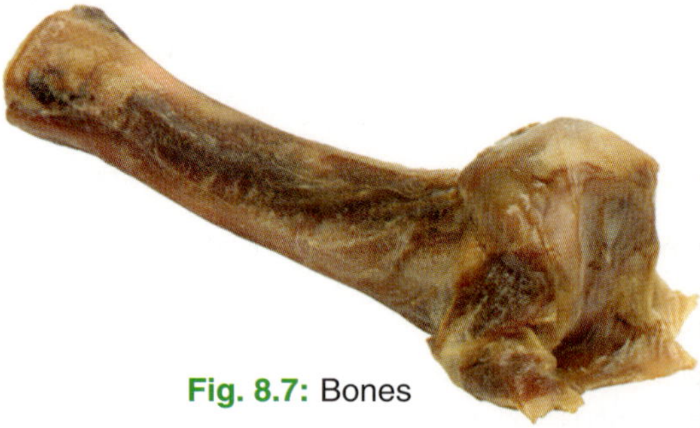

Skin with Subcutaneous Tissues

Fig. 8.7: Bones

In cases of death due to injected poisons, drugs and envenomation, site of the injection or bite must be identified. Skin around 1 cm diameter with subcutaneous tissue should be retrieved for detection of poisons and drugs in addiction and anaphylactic deaths. Sample (control) tissue from the other site must be collected for comparison. Similar tissues can also be collected in cases of electrocution at the point of entry to find out metallization with acro chemical test.

Bile

Gall bladder with bile has to be preserved by ligating the bile duct to prevent loss of bile in cases of poisoning with plant alkaloids, especially opium and opium derivatives, even when administered parenterally (enterohepatic circulation).

Blood (Fig. 8.8)

Blood acts as a carrier of poison mostly but its preservation is most essential in cases of death due to cyanide, alcohol, asphyxiants and anesthetic drugs. Blood from heart chambers or body cavities should not be collected during autopsy. At least 30 ml of blood from great vessels such as thoracic or abdominal aorta should be collected in an aseptic manner and preserved with potassium oxalate and/or sodium fluoride (for alcohol) in glass bottle.

In cases of deaths due to anesthetic agents, drug addiction deaths and death due to asphyxiants (CO, CO_2, H_2S, and FeO), blood from left ventricle must be collected and to prevent evaporation, the blood should be covered with liquid paraffin and the container should be sealed tightly.

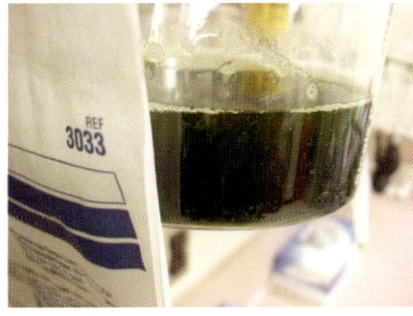

Fig. 8.8: Blood

Urine (Fig. 8.9)

Urine from the deceased must be collected to detect the presence of any toxin which is excreted through the kidney. Minimum of 30 ml of urine must be collected either by giving pressure over the bladder to collect it through the urethra or by inserting a sterile needle into the bladder to syringe it out. In both the ways care must be taken not to contaminate the urine with blood.

In living victims of poisoning or suspected poisoning 10 ml of blood and 30 ml of urine should be collected for toxicological analysis.

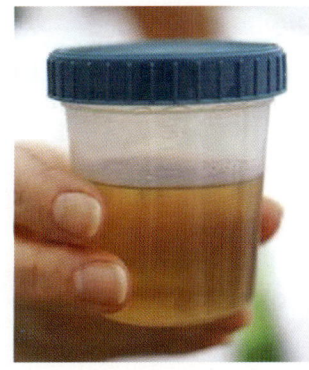

Fig. 8.9: Urine

Vitreous Humour

In cases of methyl alcohol poisoning, vitreous humour from both eyes must be collected without causing disfigurement by retracting the lateral canthus and puncturing the sclera with a wide bored needle and syringe. Minimum of 3–5 ml of fluid must be collected and must be replaced with the same amount of liquid paraffin with the same needle before withdrawal from the eyeball.

Cerebro Spinal Fluid

In cases of deaths due to alcohol, anesthetic agents, CSF should be collected during autopsy without spillage.

Lungs (Fig. 8.10)

Both the lungs must be preserved to find out the presence of inhaled poisons such as carbon monoxide, carbon dioxide, hydrogen sulphide, hydrocarbons, etc. The lungs must be harvested separately by tying the bronchus tightly and then immerse it into a jar under the coverage of liquid paraffin to prevent evaporation.

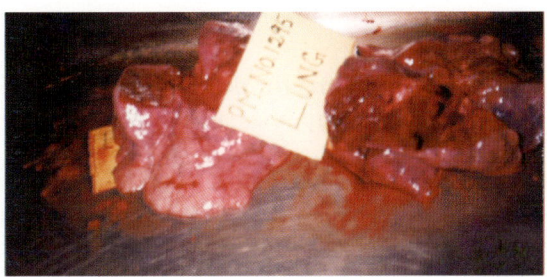

Fig. 8.10: Lungs

Soil

During exhumation soil samples from (i) above the body, (ii) right side of body, (iii) left side of body (iv) head end of the body, (v) foot end of the body, (vi) underneath the body must be collected in separate polythene bags. This helps in certain cases like arsenic poisoning, insecticidal and rodenticidal poisons. To avoid the confusion whether the poison drained from the body or imbibed from the soil into the body (arsenic), a control sample of soil should be collected well away from the grave.

Faeces

In cases of mechanical poisons such as chopped hair, glass powder and diamond dust, the faeces must be collected and examined.

Uterus (Fig. 8.11)

In cases of death due to criminal abortion, the uterus along with the entire length of vagina must be collected and preserved for toxicological analysis.

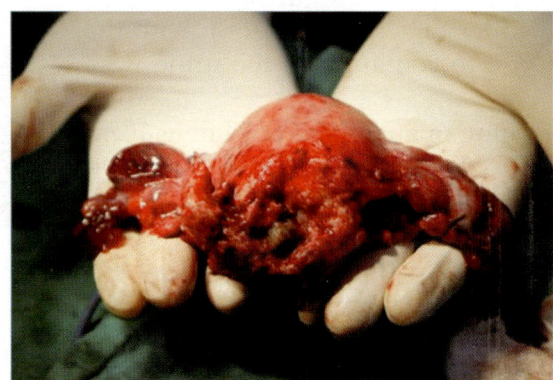

Fig. 8.11: Uterus

Swabs

In cases of poisoning death where the poison is absorbed through skin or the body orifices like middle ear and nose, the toxins can be secured with a dry, sterile cotton swab.

In cases of drowning deaths and death in conflagration, bone marrow should be collected for diatom test and carboxy-haemoglobin test respectively.

Special Cases

In unknown deaths for the purpose of confirming the identity, one long bone—preferably the femur for DNA analysis and skull for superimposition must be retrieved.

PRESERVATIVES

The samples of body tissues, organs and body fluids which are collected during the autopsy should be preserved properly in order to prevent contamination, loss and bacterial degradation. The ideal container for collecting the specimen is dry clean wide mouthed glass bottle with

1 or 2 litre capacity. The bottles should not be fully filled with preservative because adequate space should be available to accommodate the fermented gases inside the container. For this purpose suitable preservative must be added to each container only up to 1/3rd of the container and 2/3rd of the container must be left free to accommodate the gas produced by decomposition. If not, the gas will escape by lifting the lid with pressure resulting in loss of specimen also.

Common Preservatives

Rectified Spirit

Though rectified spirit is an ideal preservative, it is not being used routinely for the following reasons:

i. Availability: Not easily available and also costly
ii. Contraindications: Should not be used in cases of poisoning with alcohol, carbolic acid, phosphorous, parquet, paraldehyde, etc.
iii. Substitution: Mortuary workers may consume the rectified spirit as a substitution to the ethyl alcohol, especially in areas where prohibition is in force.

Sodium Chloride

Saturated solution of sodium chloride can be used as a preservative for all the poisons. Though sodium chloride solution is not like rectified spirit in preventing bacterial proliferation, it is easily available, cheap and there is no contraindication for its use and hence is overwhelmingly used as preservative.

Note: Sodium chloride solution should not be used to preserve tissues meant for histopathological studies.

Apart from these two common preservatives, certain special preservatives are preferred for certain toxicological analysis for better isolation of toxic principles.

Sodium Fluoride

Sodium fluoride is an ideal preservative for blood to estimate the alcohol content, since it prevents the growth of microorganisms which will ferment the blood resulting in a false report and also acts as an anticoagulant. 5 mg of sodium fluoride is necessary for 1 ml of blood.

Potassium Oxalate

It is an alternate to sodium fluoride in preservation of blood for alcohol estimation.

Glacial Acetic Acid

It is an ideal preservative for poisoning with vegetable alkaloids. Common cardiac poisons, such as oleander and aconite, poisoning the organ should be preferably preserved with this preservative in order to get a positive result.

Phenylmercuric Nitrate

This is an ideal preservative for detection of alcohol from urine.

Since urine normally contains no cellular material, it does not require any preservative. However, for preventing the loss of certain narcotic drugs and alcohol, it is preferable to be preserved with phenylmercuric nitrate.

Hydrochloric Acid

In cases of death due to gunshot injury, the gunshot residues from the hand which has fired the gun can be collected with a swab moistened with 1% HCl.

Samples that Does not Require Preservatives

Hair, bone, nails, bile (ligated gall bladder), CSF and vitreous normally does not require any preservative. Skin with underlying soft tissues dissected out from fang marks, entry wound of electrocution, and injected site of poison and insulin can also be preserved in clean glass jar without any preservative.

Never use formalin as a preservative since it is a fixative to be used for samples of histopathological examination.

PACKAGE AND LABELLING

After putting the specimen with the preservative in separate containers, each should be tightly secured and fix with wax sealing to prevent tampering. Each container should be affixed with label with the details as follows:

1. Postmortem number, date, month and year
2. Crime number and name of police station
3. Name, age and sex of the deceased.
4. Nature of the specimen with the preservative used.
5. Doctor's signature with date along with official seal.

All the containers must be rechecked to avoid wrong specimen, wrong label and unsealing. A separate container with the preservative used is also to be sent as control. All the containers should be packed in a cardboard box which should be handed over to the escort police constable immediately along with forwarding letter for transmission to the forensic laboratory after getting his specimen signature in the postmortem rough notes and also in the duplicate copy of forwarding letter. The forwarding letter should be duly filled with origin (details of the sender), and destination (receiver), number and nature of specimens, brief postmortem findings along with duplicate copy of case history (FIR) and instruct the police constable to return with the acknowledgement for receipt of the specimens at the laboratory to maintain the chain of custody. This acknowledgement must be retained with postmortem notes for further reference, if required.

Interpretation

After getting the analytical report from the Forensic Science Laboratory, it should be interpreted with the postmortem findings to give the final opinion regarding the cause of death.

Until the analytical report from the Forensic Science Laboratory is available, the opinion regarding the cause of death can be reserved.

OPINION

1. The cause of death in cases of death occurring without any medical intervention with detection of poison in all the organs can be given directly as "The deceased would appear to have died of _____ poisoning".

2. In cases where the poison could not be detected by chemical analysis the doctor should rule out possibilities of death due to causes other than poison and also to corroborate the circumstances surrounding the death, so as to give the cause of death indirectly as "The deceased would appear to have died of poisoning, but the nature of the poison could not be detected".

3. When the deceased person was treated in a hospital for a few hours or a few days for poisoning, the clinical diagnosis of death should be interpreted so as to give the cause of death as "The postmortem findings are consistent with history and clinical diagnosis of death due to _____ poisoning".

4. When the deceased was found dead and the chemical analysis is negative for poison, the doctor should give opinion based only on the circumstances after ruling out any natural disease or violence as "The postmortem findings are not inconsistent with history of death due to poisoning".

It is mandatory for the doctors who are under legal obligation in giving final opinion in the case where the cause of death is kept pending for analytical report. Before coming to a conclusion, proper interpretation with circumstances and analytical report with postmortem finding is most essential and important. The doctor should be able to categorize whether the poison is solely responsible in causing death (conclusive cause) or the poison has contributed to death (contributory cause) or the poison has no role in death (some other disease or trauma).

Based on the above facts, the opinion of the doctor will determine the further course of investigation. Hence the knowledge of forensic toxicology is most important to every doctor.

NEGATIVE CHEMICAL ANALYSIS REPORT

The chemical analysis need not detect the poison always because of the following reasons:

1. Complete evacuation through vomit
2. Complete excretion through kidneys or bowel.
3. Complete metabolisation in the body.
4. Complete evaporation through lungs.
5. Insufficient quantity of poison in the sample.
6. Improper selection of tissues.
7. Improper preservation of samples.
8. Undue delay in analyzing the samples.
9. Improper tests carried out.
10. Denaturation or deterioration due to decomposition.
11. No sensitive test to detect the poison.
12. Poison may be converted into ionic components of body tissues, e.g. snake venom, insulin, etc.

9

Forensic Spotters

BASIC CONCEPT IN IDENTIFICATION OF SPOTTERS

It is an universal fact that every object or article is characterised by its physical peculiarities or features. These physical appearances are unique to that particular object alone. The physical appearance is helpful to fix the identity of that particular object.

Before naming the spotter the important physical features should be given as a proof of identification. After establishing the positive identity the other details should be answered as per the requirement mentioned.

Stomach Wash Tube

A flexible but non-collapsible linear rubber tube 1.5 metre long and 1.25 cm in diameter. One end is fitted with a funnel, the other end is blunt and round with central and peripheral holes. Near the funnel end an elliptical dilatation (suction bulb) is also present. This is stomach wash tube or gastric lavage tube (Fig. 9.1).

Uses: To evacuate the unabsorbed ingested poison.

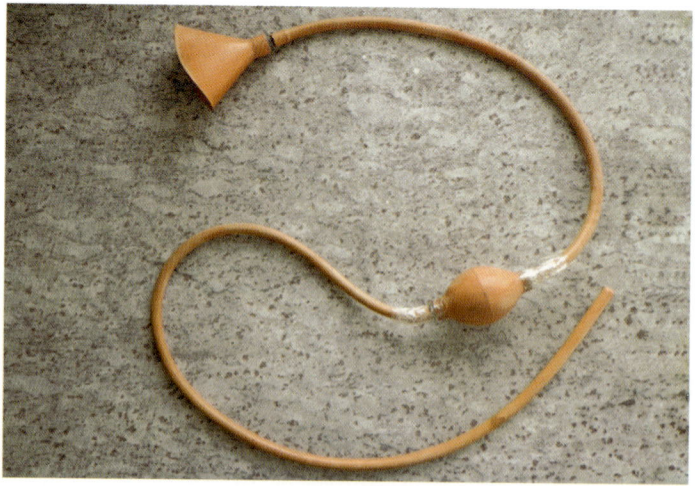

Fig. 9.1: Stomach wash tube

Contraindications for stomach wash:

1. Corrosive poisons (except carbolic acid)
2. Convulsions
3. Coma
4. Cirrhosis of liver (oesophageal varices)
5. Cold (hypothermia)
6. Congestive cardiac failure
7. Children (Ryle's tube)
8. Child birth (pregnancy)
9. Hydrocarbons (volatile poisons)

Criminal Use

1. Postmortem poisoning to mislead investigation.
2. Strangulation

Medicolegal Importance

Death can be prevented by timely evacuation of unabsorbed poison from the stomach.

CORROSIVE POISONS

It is postmortem specimen of stomach.

The mucosa of the stomach is swollen, oedematous, tarry black in colour and friable in nature.

This is a specimen of stomach in sulphuric acid poisoning (Fig. 9.2).

Mechanism of Action of Sulphuric Acid

Local action only: Sulphuric acid is a corrosive poison causing destruction and dehydration of gastric mucosa with carbonisation. It causes coagulation necrosis. Perforation is common.

Fig. 9.2: Specimen of stomach in sulphuric acid poisoning

Medicolegal Importance

1. Suicide is common
2. Accident is also possible
3. Homicide is rare
4. Vitriolage is common

Carbolic Acid

Dark brown (coffee brown) watery fluid emitting the characteristic odour of phenol. The given specimen is carbolic acid (Fig. 9.3) which is a corrosive poison.

Mode of Action

1. Local: Corrosion of stomach mucosa which becomes thick and hardened like a leather bag.
2. Systemic: Depression of the central nervous system. Pinpoint pupil, coma, convulsions and death.

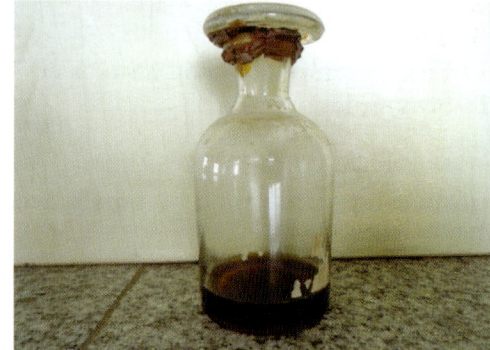

Medicolegal Importance

1. Suicide is common
2. Accidental poison is not uncommon
3. Homicide never
4. Abortifacient

Fig. 9.3: Carbolic acid

Carboluria: Excretion of by-products of carbolic acid (hydroquinone and pyrocatechol) in the urine is known as carboluria. The freshly voided urine is colourless but it turns into smoky green on exposure due to further oxidation of carbolic acid and its by-products.

Oxalic Acid

White prismatic crystalline powder, bitter in taste with no odour resembling table salt or epsom salt. The given specimen is oxalic acid (Fig. 9.4) which is a corrosive poison.

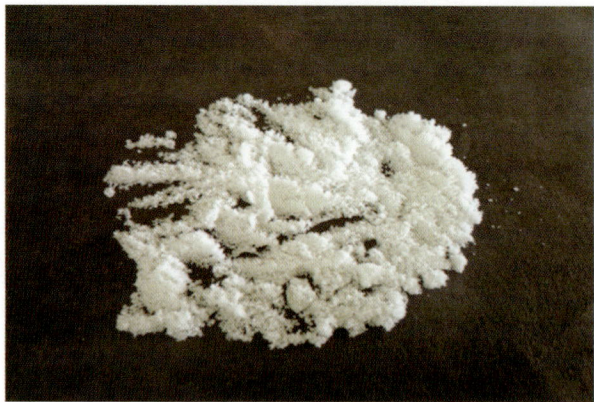

Fig. 9.4: Oxalic acid

Mode of Action

1. Local: Corrosion of the stomach mucosa relatively less severe than other corrosive acids.
2. Systemic: Combines with serum calcium causing severe hypocalcemia — tetany.

Antidote

1. Calcium lactate for stomach wash
2. Calcium gluconate IV for absorbed poison.

Medicolegal Importance

1. Accidental poisoning is common
2. Suicide and homicide are rare
3. Forgery of documents

Oxaluria: Presence of calcium oxalate crystals in urine is known as oxaluria.

IRRITANT POISONS

Inorganic Irritant Poison

(Metallic irritants)

Arsenic

A dull white amorphous powder with no odour or taste. The given specimen is arsenic tri-oxide or white arsenic (Fig. 9.5) which is a metallic irritant poison.

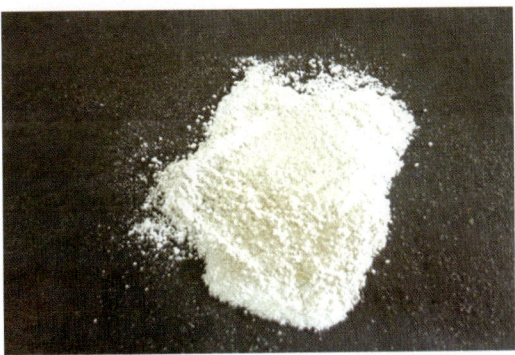

Fig. 9.5: White arsenic

Mode of Action

Systemic: Combines with sulphydryl group of cytochrome enzymes affecting the cellular metabolism and damage of blood vessels.

Local: Causes irritation of stomach mucosa and increases the permeability of intestinal mucosa with inflammatory necrosis resulting in vomiting and cholera-like diarrhoea.

Antidote

1. Stomach wash with freshly prepared ferric hydroxide solution
2. Dimercaprol IM, DMSA (succimer) orally, or DMPS (unithiol) orally.

Medicolegal Importance

1. It is an ideal homicidal poison.
2. Accidental poisoning is common as contaminant of food and beverages.
3. Suicide is rare.

Lead Tetroxide or Red Lead

Scarlet red sprinkling powder with no odour or taste. This is the specimen of lead tetroxide or red lead (vermillion) (Fig. 9.6) which is a metallic irritant poison.

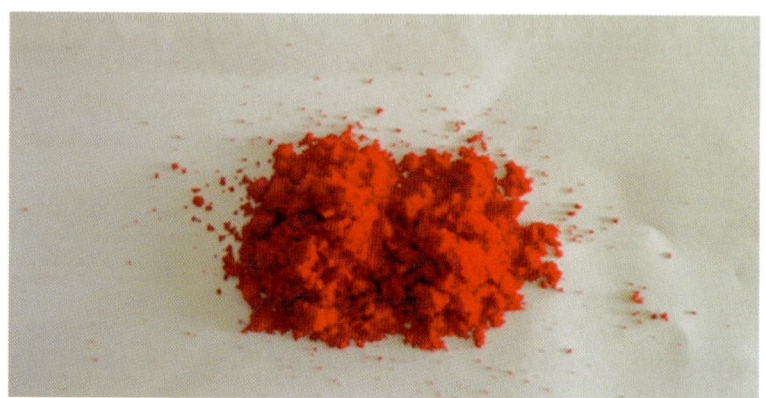

Fig. 9.6: Lead tetroxide

Mechanism of Action

Local action: Irritant action

Systemic: Combines with sulphydryl group of enzymes and interferes with metabolism, inhibits haeme synthesis and increased accumulation of delta amino leuvulinic acid and protoporphyrin in blood and urine.

Antidote

1. Stomach wash with sodium or magnesium sulphate.
2. Dimercaprol (BAL) and EDTA.

Medicolegal Importance

1. Accidental poisoning is common because of wide industrial use.
2. Suicide and homicide rare.
3. Abortifacient.
4. Chronic poisoning (plumbism) with lead is more common than acute poisoning.

Copper

Bluish or bluish green glistening crystalline powder with metallic taste and no odour. This specimen is copper sulphate (Fig. 9.7) which is a metallic irritant poison.

Mode of Action

Local: Irritant haemorrhagic gastritis

Systemic: Powerful enzyme inhibitor induces hemolysis, centri lobular necrosis of liver with biliary stasis and renal tubular necrosis.

Antidote

1. Unabsorbed: Stomach wash with potassium ferrocyanide solution results in formation of cupric cyanide which is harmless.
2. Absorbed (systemic):
    i. Penicillamine 20–30 mg/kg in divided dose orally and/or
    ii. BAL.

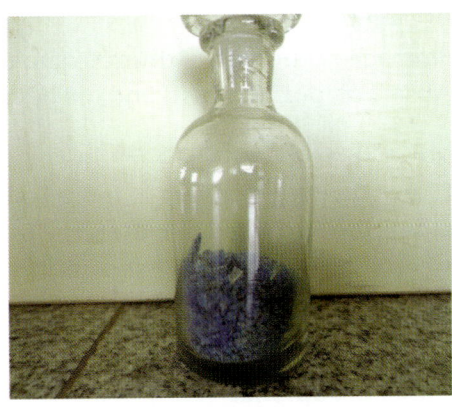

Fig. 9.7: Copper sulphate

Medicolegal Importance

1. Suicide is common with copper sulphate
2. Accidental poison is possible due to occupational exposure.
3. Homicide can never occur.
4. Abortifacient.

Mercury

Brick red crystalline powder with no odour. The specimen is mercuric sulphide (Fig. 9.8) which is a metallic irritant poison.

Mode of Action

Local: Gastric irritation

Systemic: Combines with sulphydryl radical of enzymes and affects kidneys (renal tubular necrosis) and causes liver damage.

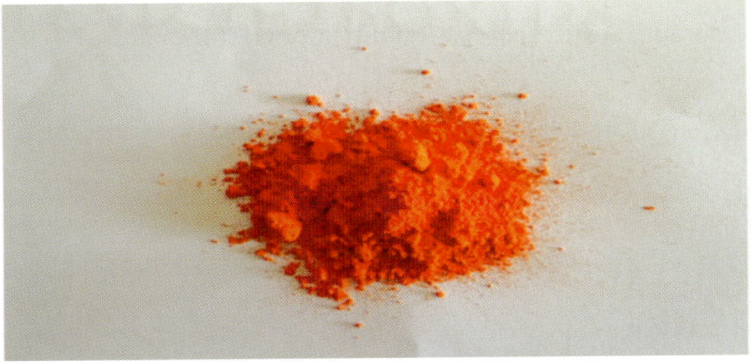

Fig. 9.8: Mercuric sulphide

Antidote

Stomach wash with sodium formaldehyde sulphoxylate solution.
Absorbed poison: BAL and/or penicillamine

Medicolegal Importance

1. Accidental poisoning is more common.
2. Suicide and homicide are very rare.

Organic Irritant Poisons

Vegetable Irritant Poisons

Abrus precatorius

Egg or oval-shaped hard seed, scarlet red in colour with a dark spot. This is the seed of *Abrus precatorius* (Fig. 9.9) which is a vegetable irritant poison.

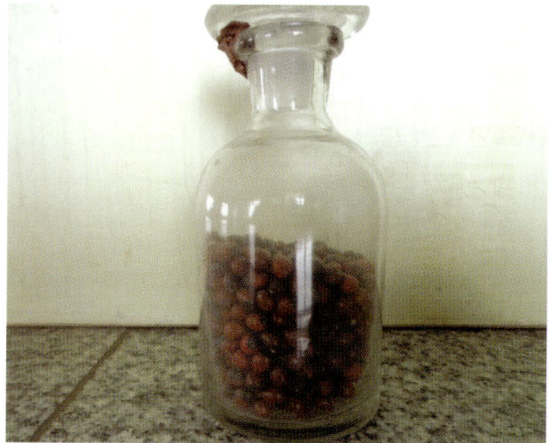

Fig. 9.9: Seed of *Abrus precatorius*—vegetable irritant poison

Toxic Principles

Abrin, abrine and abralin. Abrin is a toxalbumin, a powerful toxin.

Mode of Action

It causes agglutination, haemolysis and vascular injury.

Antidote

Antiabrin

Medicolegal Importance

1. Ideal cattle poison (sui)
2. Accidental poison common among children
3. Suicide and homicide are rare.

Ricinus communis

Oval-shaped brownish seed with white dots with a nose-like projection at one end. The outer shell is hard harbouring a soft white pulp and on pressure it yields an oily fluid. This is seed of *Ricinus communis* or castor bean (Fig. 9.10) which is a vegetable irritant poison.

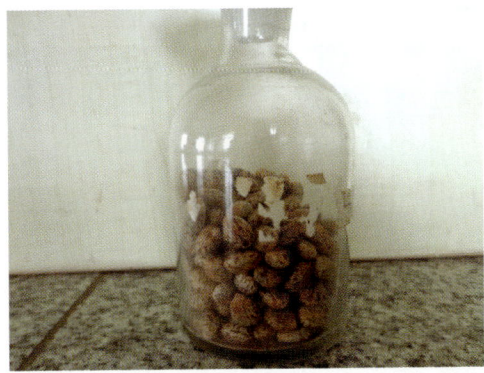

Fig. 9.10: Seed of *Ricinus communis*—vegetable irritant poison

Active Principle

Ricin which is a toxalbumin present in the press cake only and not in the oil.

Mode of Action

Ricin being a toxalbumin causes lysis and agglutination of red cells and antibody production.

Medicolegal Importance

1. Accidental poison may occur among children.
2. Weapon of bio-terrorism.
3. Suicide and homicide are rare.

Semecarpus Anacardium

Brownish black, hard, kidney-shaped, dry shrivelled seed. This is the specimen of *Semecarpus anacardium* or marking nut (Fig. 9.11) which is a vegetable irritant poison.

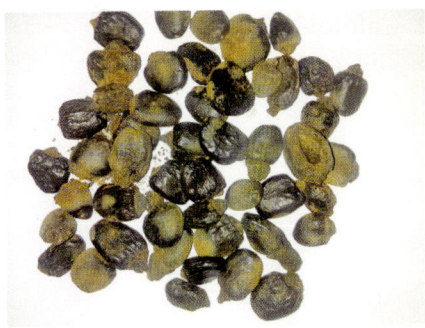

Fig. 9.11: Seed of *Semecarpus anacardium* —vegetable irritant poison

Toxic Principles

1. Semecarpol
2. Bhilawanol

Mode of Action

Powerful vesicant causes painful blisters over the skin and mucosa and causes toxic myocarditis.

Medicolegal Importance

1. Accidental poison may occur in quackery medicine
2. Artificial bruise by malingerers
3. Abortifacient.

Calotropis

A green plant grows wildly in wasteland. The leaves are broad, arranged as opposite pairs in the stem. On incision of the leaves or the stem it yields an acrid milky juice. Flowers are seen as terminal clusters, purple in colour and boat-shaped green fruit. This is a specimen of calotropis plant (*Calotropis gigantea* (Fig. 9.12) which is a vegetable irritant poison).

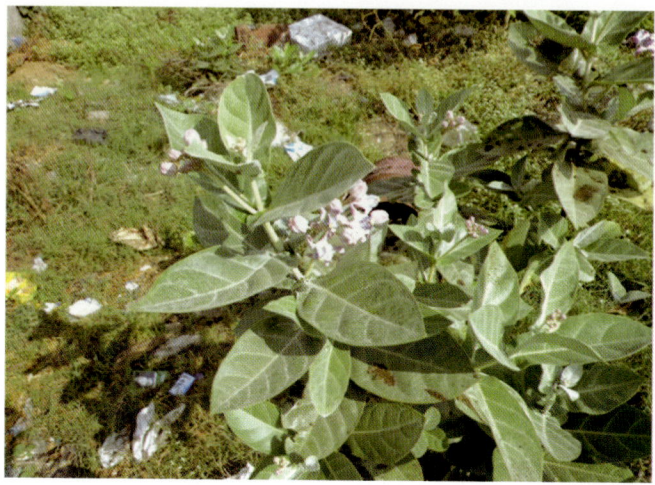

Fig. 9.12: *Calotropis gigantea*—vegetable irritant poison

Toxic Principles

1. Calotropin
2. Calotoxin
3. Gigantin
4. Usharin

Mode of Action

Vesication over skin and mucosa and toxic effect on heart muscles and brain.

Medicolegal Importance

1. Abortifacient
2. Infanticide
3. Cattle poisoning

Animal poisons

Cobra

A linear cylindrical limbless animal having a head, body and tail. The tail is short, stout and blunt. The body is longer, wheatish in colour covered with scales. The head is oval in shape with a pair of nostrils and rounded eyes. The neck is distended with a spectacle mark over the hood. This is the specimen of common cobra (Fig. 9.13).

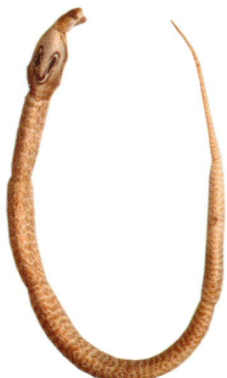

Fig. 9.13: Cobra

Toxic Principles

The venom secreted by the parotid salivary gland is a mixture of toxic protein and peptides.

Mode of Action

Neurotoxin: Affecting the nervous system causing paralysis of respiratory centre.

Antidote

Polyvalent antisnake venom

Medicolegal Importance

1. Accidental bite is very common
2. Homicide rare
3. Suicide never preferred.

Common Krait

Elongated cylindrical limbless animal with head, body and tail; steel black in colour with alternate thin white transparent band seen from neck to tail. This is the specimen of common krait (Fig. 9.14).

Toxic Principle

Neurotoxic venom, a complex mixture of lytic proteins and peptides.

Mode of Action

Powerful neurotoxic poison which paralyses the nervous system.

Antidote

Polyvalent antisnake venom.

Medicolegal Importance

1. Accidental bite is very common.
2. Homicide and suicide are very rare.

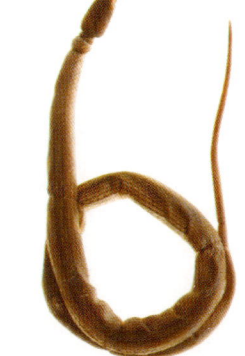

Fig. 9.14: Common krait

Viper

A stout elongated limbless animal with a triangular head, a distinct neck, body and blunt tail; brownish in colour. Eyes are vertical. A chain of black circular band on the body with semicircular band on either side over the body. This is the specimen of russel viper (Fig. 9.15).

Toxic Principle

Haemotoxic venom, a complex mixture of lytic proteins and peptides.

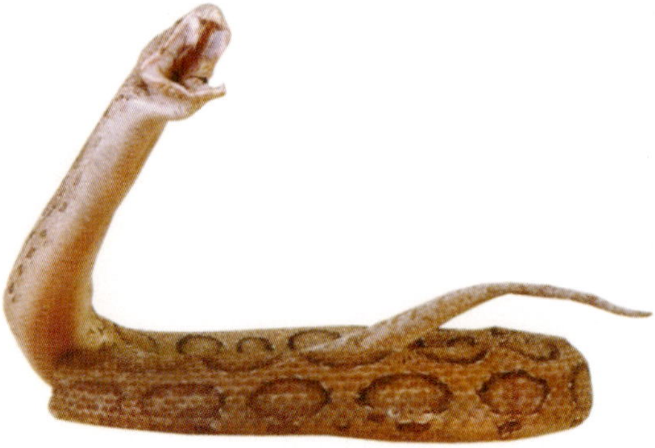

Mode of Action

Local: Spreading cellulitis
Systemic: Hemolytic action resulting in coagulation disorder and hemolysis with acute tubular necrosis.

Antidote

Polyvalent antisnake venom.

Fig. 9.15: Russel viper

Medicolegal Importance

1. Accidental bite is very common.
2. Homicide and suicide are very rare.

Scorpion

A headless ugliest animal having cephalothorax and abdomen with six-segmented tail, a pair of claw in front and four pairs of legs on sides; brownish red in colour. The terminal segment of tail is enlarged like a bulb called telson provided with the stinger which is connected with the venom gland. This is a specimen of scorpion (Fig. 9.16).

Toxic Principle

The venom is a complex mixture of lytic protein which acts like a toxalbumin.

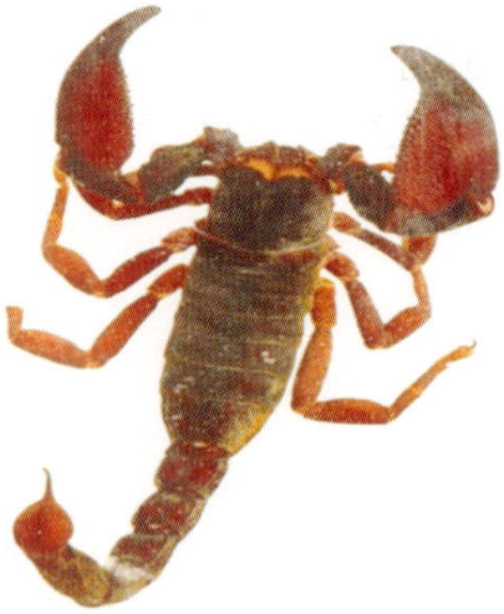

Mode of Action

Neurotoxic, hemolytic and cardiotoxic poison.

Medicolegal Importance

1. Accidental sting is very common.
2. Homicide and suicide are very very rare.

Fig. 9.16: Scorpion

NEUROTOXIC POISONS

Papaverum somniferum

It is a green plant, cultivation of which requires government license. The juice obtained by incision made on the unripe fruit yields opium which on drying becomes a solid latex containing a variety of alkaloids. The riped fruit is brownish yellow in colour and contains fine granular seeds (kaskas) which is non-poisonous.

Active Principle

The alkaloids in the crude opium are broadly classified as phenanthrene group and isoquinoline group.

Phenanthrene Group

Morphine
Codeine
Thebaine

Isoquinoline Group

Papaverine
Narcotin
Narceine

Mode of Action

CNS depression by combining with specific receptors kappa, delta and mu in the brain. Its analgesic effect is being utilised to kill pain along with undue desire to sleep, a side effect.

Medicolegal Importance

1. Powerful drug of addiction
2. Accidental death is more common
3. Suicide and homicide are rare

Deliriant

Datura

A small green plant with broad leaves, bell-shaped single flower, green spherical fruit with sharp spikes. This is *Datura niger* (purple flower) or *Datura alba* (white flower) (Fig. 9.17) which is a deliriant poison.

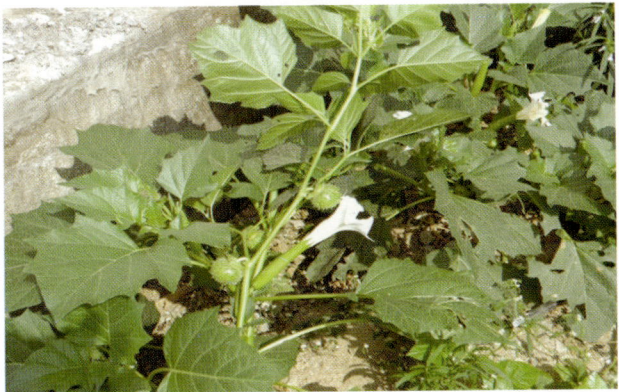

Fig. 9.17: Datura

Toxic Principles

Hyoscine, hyoscyamine and traces of atropine

Mode of Action

Blocks the acetyl choline receptor. Stimulates the central nervous system initially by sympathomimetic action followed by depression and atropine stimulates the heart by its vagolytic effect.

Antidote

Neostigmine/prostigmine or pilocarpine

Medicolegal Importance

1. It is an ideal stupefier to facilitate kidnapping, rape and robbery.
2. Death is rare usually due to accidental poisoning.

Spinal Poison

Strychnos nux-vomica

Ash grey-coloured disc-shaped hard concavo-convex seed covered with soft fine strands. This is the specimen of *Strychnos nux-vomica* (Fig. 9.18) which is a convulsive poison.

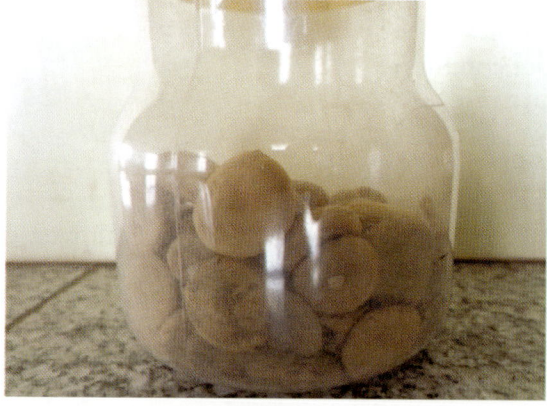

Fig. 9.18: *Strychnos nux-vomica*

Toxic Principles

Strychnine and brucine

Mode of Action

Acts on the anterior horn cells of the spinal cord accentuating the spinal reflex swiftly even with slightest stimulus.

Antidote

Ultra short acting barbiturate (pentathol sodium IV)

Medicolegal Importance

1. Accidental poison may occur due to inadvertent use in native medicine.
2. Ideal arrow poison for hunting.

CARDIAC POISONS

Aconite

Conical-shaped dry root with tapering end, dark brown in colour with shrivelled longitudinal wrinkles. This is the specimen of aconite root (Fig. 9.19) which is a cardiac poison.

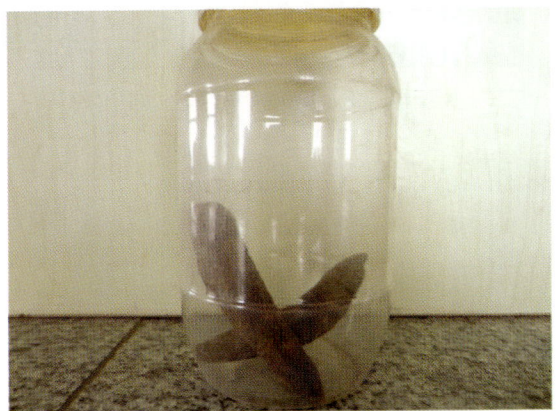

Fig. 9.19: Aconite root

Toxic Principles

Aconitine, pseudoaconitine and aconine

Mode of Action

Initial stimulation of sensory and motor nerve endings followed by paralysis of medullary centres and profound cardiac arrhythmias.

Antidote

No specific antidote. Atropine can be given to revert the cardiac arrhythmias.

Medicolegal Importance

1. Accidental poisoning is common.
2. Homicidal is unusual but possible.
3. Suicide rare.
4. Ideal arrow poison

Cerebra thevetia

A green plant with leaves which is light green, soft and lanceolate in shape. The flowers are single, yellow in colour and bell-shaped. Green spherical fruits contain triangular seeds. This is the specimen of *Cerebra thevetia* or yellow oleander plant (Fig. 9.20) which is a cardiac poison.

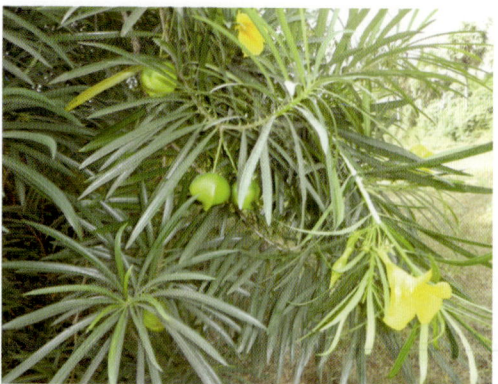

Fig. 9.20: *Cerebra thevetia*

Toxic Principles

Cerebrin, thevetin, thevetoxin, ruvoside and peruvoside.

Mode of Action

Local: Gastric irritation
Systemic: Heart block

Antidote

No specific antidote

Medicolegal Importance

1. Suicide is common
2. Abortifacient
3. Cattle poison
4. Homicide is rare

Nerium odorum

A green plant. The leaves are dark green in colour, thick and fleshy in consistency and lanceolate in shape. The flowers are pink in colour and seen as terminal clusters. This is the specimen of *Nerium odorum* or pink oleander (Fig. 9.21) which is a cardiac poison.

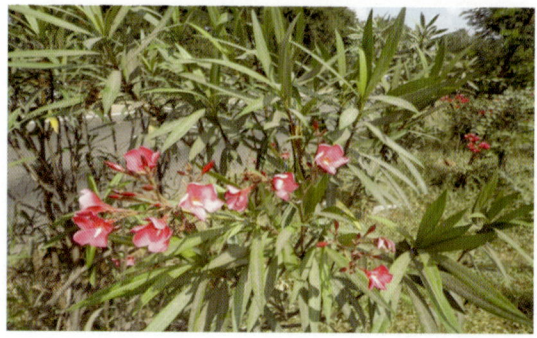

Fig. 9.21: *Nerium odorum*

Toxic Principles

Nerine
Oleandrine

Mode of Action

Local: Gastric irritation
Systemic: Heart block

Antidote

No specific antidote

Medicolegal Importance

1. Suicide is common
2. Abortifacient
3. Cattle poison
4. Homicide is rare

Ricinus communis

Plant with pinkish stem and green leaves which are broad like palm with spread out fingers. Fruits are green in colour covered with soft projections which contains two or more brown seeds.

This is a specimen of *Ricinus communis* or castor plant which is a vegetable irritant poison.

Toxic Principles

Ricin (Fig. 9.22), which is a toxalbumin present abundantly in the seeds.

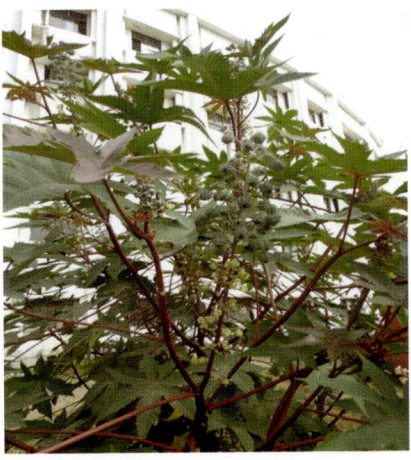

Fig. 9.22: *Ricinus communis*

Mode of Action

The pollen on contact causes allergic rhinitis and conjunctivitis. Ricin being a toxalbumin causes bleeding tendency due to increased vascular permeability, haemolysis and haemagglutination.

Medicolegal Importance

1. Accident is more common
2. Suicide and homicide are very rare.

WEAPONS

Lathi

A linear 3–4 feet long cylindrical, non-flexible stick with nodes and internodes. The proximal end fitted with a leather strap with a loop and the distal end is also covered with a leather strap. This specimen is lathi (Fig. 9.23) made of bamboo which is a light blunt weapon.

Possible Injuries

Abrasion, contusion, laceration and fracture of small bones of the limbs. The contusion caused by this implement looks like tram line-patterned contusion.

Medicolegal Importance

It is a dangerous weapon.

Hammer

A blackish rectangular heavy metallic object having two ends and four surfaces fitted with a wooden handle through a central hole. This is a hammer (Fig. 9.24) which is a moderately heavy blunt weapon.

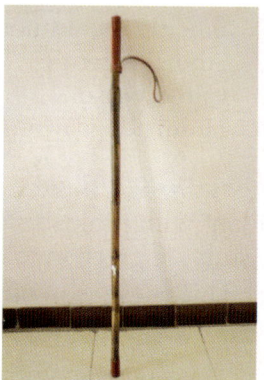

Fig. 9.23: Lathi

Possible Injuries

Abrasion, contusion, laceration and fracture of bones. It causes a depressed fracture over the vault of skull almost equal to the size and shape of the striking end, hence it is called fracture-a-la-signature.

Medicolegal Importance

1. It is a dangerous weapon
2. Homicide is possible
3. Accident can occur
4. Suicide is rare

Rope

A white linear collapsible object made from twisted cotton threads. This is cotton rope (Fig. 9.25), a flexible blunt implement.

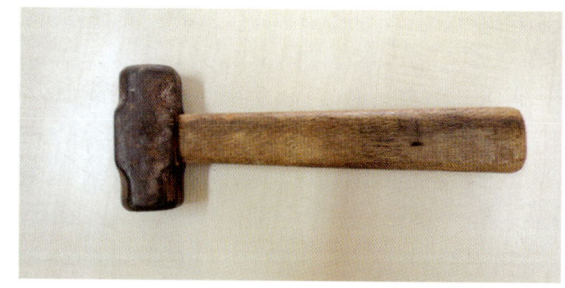

Fig. 9.24: Hammer

Possible Injuries

Abrasion, contusion

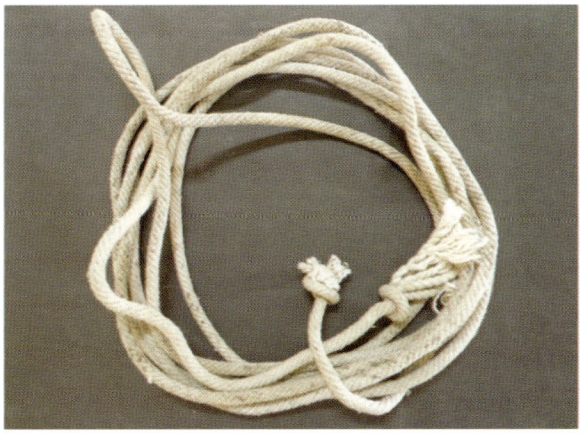

Fig. 9.25: Rope

Medicolegal Importance

1. Used to commit suicide by hanging
2. Homicidal strangulation is common and suicidal strangulation (spanish windlass) is also possible.
3. Rendering the victims incapable to resist the assailant by binding the limbs.

Knife

A flat metallic plate designed to have two ends, two edges and two surfaces. The distal end gradually tapering to a sharp tip and the proximal end is fitted with a green plastic handle. One edge is sharpened and the other edge is blunt. This is a kitchen knife (Fig. 9.26) which is a light weight sharp weapon.

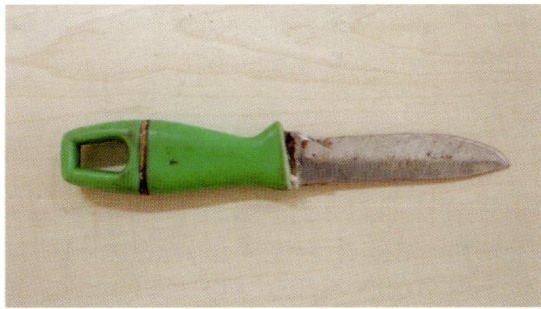

Fig. 9.26: Knife

Possible Injuries

Tip: Scratch, punctured wound (stab)
Sharp edge: Incised wound
Blunt edge and handle: Abrasion, contusion and laceration

Medicolegal Importance

It is a dangerous weapon.
Death due to homicide and suicide is possible.
Accidental death is rare.

Bitchuva

A flat metallic blade designed to have two ends, two edges and two surfaces. The distal end gradually tapering to a sharp tip and the proximal end is fitted with a white plastic handle. Both edges are sharp but the body is curved at two points. This is bitchuva (Fig. 9.27), a double-edged curved light weapon.

Possible Injuries

Tip: Scratch, stab—length of the stab is longer than the breadth of the weapon because of the curvature.
Edges: Incised wound
Handle: Abrasion, contusion, laceration.

Medicolegal Importance

1. It is a dangerous weapon.
2. Homicide is common
3. Suicide is possible
4. Accident—never.

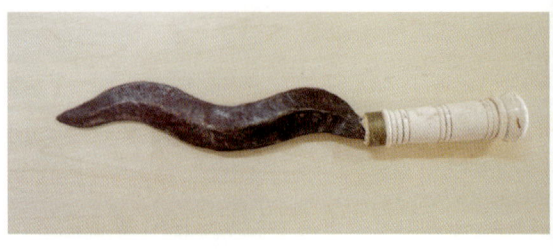

Fig. 9.27: Bitchuva

Sickle

A thick flat and elongated metal designed to have two ends, two edges and two surfaces. One end is fitted with a wooden handle and the other end is curved and tapering to a sharp tip. The curved edge is sharp and the other edge is blunt. The surfaces are smooth. Since it resembles sickle cell, it is called sickle (Fig. 9.28) which is a moderately heavy cutting weapon.

Possible Injuries

Tip: Scratch and stab
Sharp end: Incised wound, amputation and decapitation.
Blunt edge and handle: Abrasion, contusion, laceration and fracture.

Medicolegal Importance

1. It is a dangerous weapon.
2. Homicide is common.
3. Suicide is rare.
4. Accident is not possible.

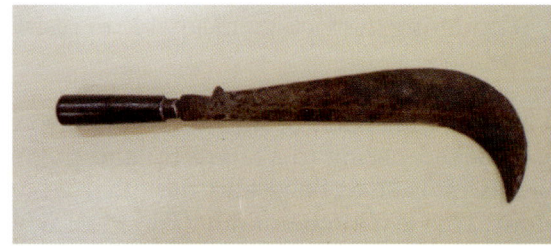

Fig. 9.28: Sickle

Serrated Sickle

A thin flat curved metallic instrument designed to have two ends, two edges and two surfaces. One end is fitted with a wooden handle and the other end is curved and tapering to a sharp tip. One edge is blunt and the other end is sharp made into fine saw tooth-like projections. The surfaces are smooth. Because of the shape and serration it is serrated sickle (Fig. 9.29), which is a moderately heavy cutting weapon.

Possible Injuries

Tip: Scratch and stab
Sharp edge: Incised wound with irregular wound margin and decapitation.
Blunt edge and handle: Abrasion, contusion, laceration and fracture.

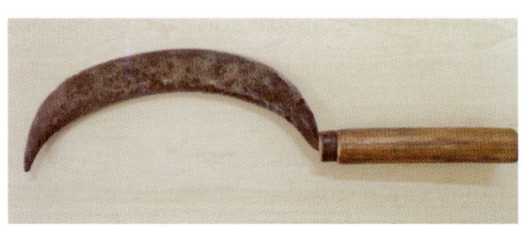

Fig. 9.29: Serrated sickle

Medicolegal Importance

It is a dangerous weapon.

Butcher's Knife

It is a heavy flat, thick metallic object designed to have two ends, two edges, two surfaces. One end is fitted with a wooden handle and the other end is broad and slightly curved. One edge is sharp and the other end is blunt and flat with slight upward curve at the end. This is a heavy cutting weapon commonly used by butchers. It is called butcher's knife (Fig. 9.30).

Possible Injuries

Sharp end: Incised wound or gaping incised wound and chop wound, decapitation and amputation.

Blunt edge: Abrasion, contusion, laceration and fracture.

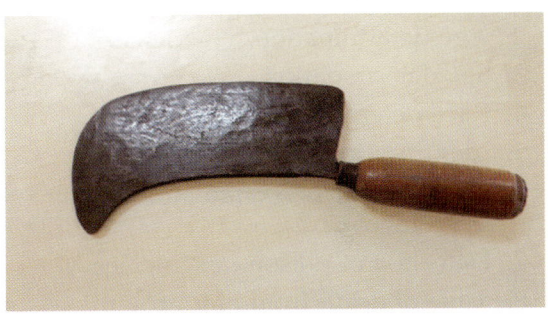

Medicolegal Importance

1. It is a dangerous weapon.
2. Homicide is common.
3. Suicide is rare.
4. Accident is rare.

Fig. 9.30: Butcher's knife

Cartridge

A short red colour empty paper tube fitted with a metallic cap. Over the centre of the metal base, percussion cap is attached. The other end is open. This is a fired shot shell or empty cartridge of a shot gun. (Fig. 9.31).

Diagram of longitudinal section of unfired shot shell with its components is given in Fig. 9.32.

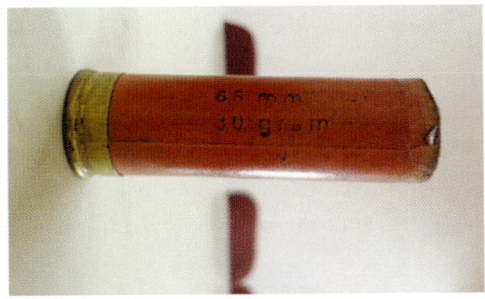

Fig. 9.31: Cartridge

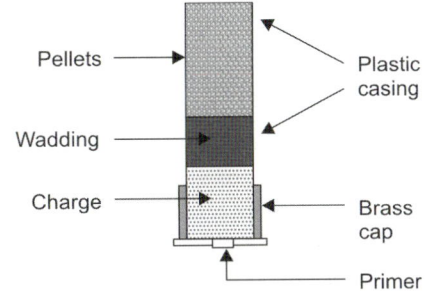

Fig. 9.32: Unfired shot sheel

Medicolegal Importance

1. It is a lethal weapon.
2. Homicide is common, accident is not uncommon.
3. Suicide is rare.

FORENSIC MICROSCOPY

Hair

The slide shows a linear structure having a rounded base (root), a long body (shaft) and tapering terminal (tip). The shaft shows an outer wavy pattern (cuticle), middle dark area (cortex) and innermost hypodense irregular area (medulla). The specimen is identified as hair (Fig. 9.33).

Medicolegal Importance

Useful in:

1. Species identification.
2. Age determination.
3. Sex determination.
4. Race determination
5. Identification of accused in rape.
6. Identification of weapon in assault or vehicle in accident cases.
7. Detection of poison (arsenic, lead).
8. Time of death from hair growth.
9. DNA analysis.
10. Hair is not affected by decomposition, hence it is a long-lasting evidence of human tissue useful in forensic identification.

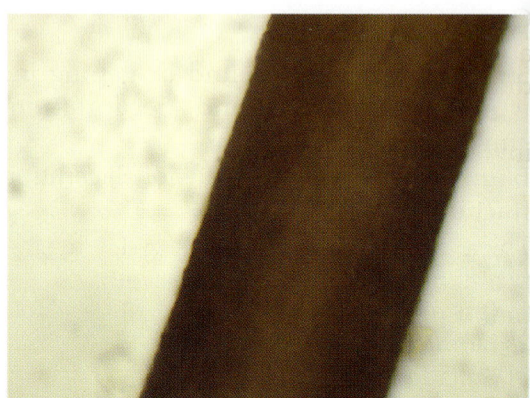

Fig. 9.33: Hair

Diatom

The slide shows a boat-shaped, cylindrical and an elliptical-shaped unicellular bodies having a thick outer wall. These are diatoms (Fig. 9.34), which are unicellular bodies found in fresh, sea and brackish water. The thick wall is made up of silica, which is acid resistant. They are of different shapes and sizes, vary in different places and season. The diatom enters into the body through inhaled water and carried to all parts of the body by circulation in antemortem drowning. This can be demonstrated by acid digestion.

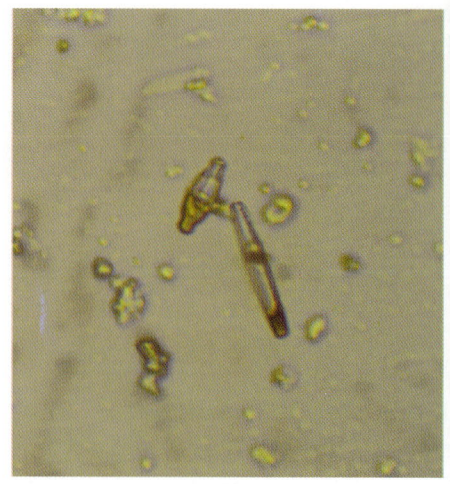

Medicolegal Importance

1. To differentiate antemortem drowning from postmortem drowning.
2. To find out the place of drowning.
3. To find out the season of drowning.
4. Superior to other chemical tests as the diatom is not affected by decomposition.

Fig. 9.34: Diatom

FORENSIC PHOTOGRAPHY

Hit and Run Case

This photo shows a male dead body in a prone position. Zigzag wavy patterned purplish blue discoloration obliquely seen across the back of chest and abdomen with intervening intact skin. This is a patterned contusion caused by tread pattern of heavy vehicle tyre (Fig. 9.35).

Medicolegal Importance

Cause of death: It is a proof of hit and run over by a heavy vehicle on the victim resulting in death due to crush injury chest and abdomen.

From tyre tread pattern on the body, the vehicle involved can be identified.

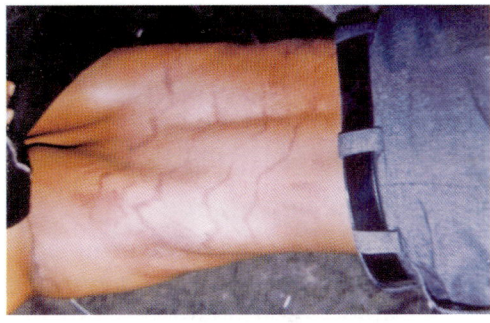

Fig. 9.35: Forensic photography of hit and run case

Drowning

This photo shows a body of a male lying in supine position. There is fine white froth exuding from the nose and mouth. Pale brown fine sand particles also seen over the face, neck and chest. Hence it is identified as a victim of drowning (Fig. 9.36).

The inhaled water, bronchial secretions and air in the lung churned in trachea and bronchi to form fine tenacious froth which exudes through nose and mouth.

Medicolegal Importance

Fine froth over the nose and mouth of a body recovered from water is the surest sign of antemortem drowning irrespective of suicidal, homicidal or accidental manner.

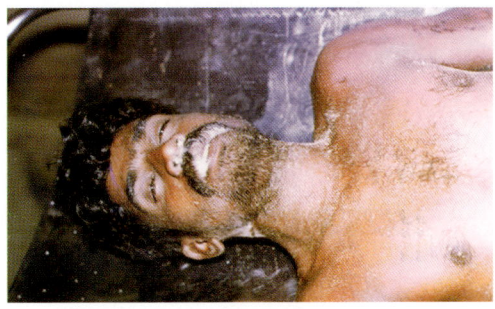

Fig. 9.36: Forensic photography of drowning

Throttling

This photo shows the body of a female lying on her back with extended neck. Multiple crescentric abrasions of varying sizes seen below the chin, over left mandibular region and front of neck. As these abrasions approximately equalising the size and shape of finger nails, it is identified as a victim of throttling (Fig. 9.37).

Medicolegal Importance

1. Crescentric abrasions are caused by tucking of nails into epidermis (patterned abrasions).
2. It is a typical sign of manual strangulation.
3. Epithelial debris can be detected from the assailant (Locard's principle of exchange).

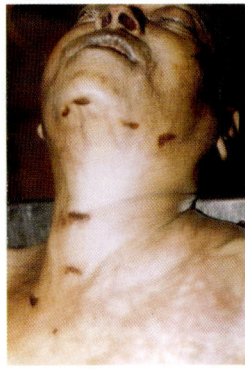

Fig. 9.37: Forensic photography of throttling

Gunshot

Photo of a male body exposing front of left side of chest. There is a circular punctured wound between left nipple and axilla. Immediately around the punctured wound is a pale zone surrounded by a blackish zone. No oozing of blood or protrusion of tissues. It is entry wound of gunshot. (Fig. 9.38)

Mechanism: The pale zone around the punctured wound is due to loss of epidermis by the spin of the penetrating bullet nooze and the black zone around it is due to the wiped dirt from the body of the bullet.

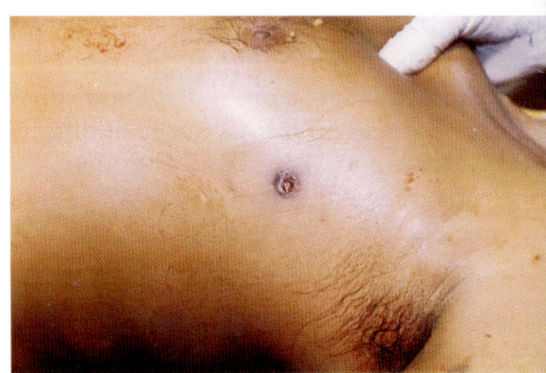

Medicolegal Importance

1. Range of firing can be determined.
2. Direction of firing can be determined.
3. Positional relationship of the victim and assailant can be ascertained.
4. The fire arm which discharges the shot can be identified.
5. Motive of the assailant can be presumed.

Fig. 9.38: Forensic photography of gunshot

Defence Wounds

Photo of a male body exposing the injured left forearm. There is an incised wound 7cm × 1cm × muscle deep over the middle third of outer aspect and the left hand is severed at the level of the wrist. The severed hand is attached with the tag of skin over the radial border. The wounds are defence wounds (Fig. 9.39).

Mechanism: Wound sustained during the instinctive reaction of the victim to defend the attack.

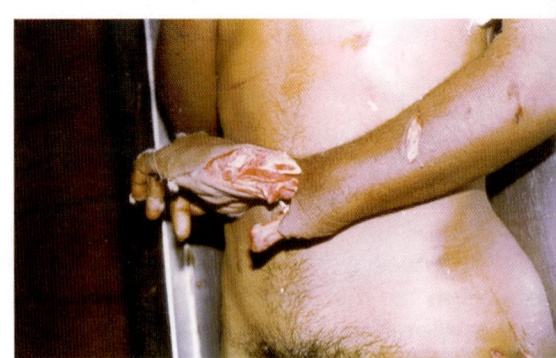

Medicolegal Importance

1. Defence wounds are commonly seen in assault.
2. It is a proof of antemortem wound.
3. Type of wound reflects the type of force.
4. Site of injury reflects the nature of the defender either to hold off the weapon or guard off the body part.

Fig. 9.39: Forensic photography of defence wound

Bibliography

1. *Detection of Human Remains*, 2 edn by Edward W Killam.
2. *Sexual Assault: The Medicolegal Examination* by Sharon R Crowby RN, MN PHN.
3. *Forensic Radiology* by KT Evans, B Knight, DK Whittaker.
4. *Sex-Related Homicide and Death Investigation Practical and Clinical Perspectives* by Vermon J Geberth.
5. *Fundamentals of Forensic Science* by Max Herick, Jay Siegel, 2006.
6. *Forensic Pathology of Trauma* by Michael J Shkrum, David A Ramsay, 2007.
7. *Forensic Pathology* by Dominick J, Di Maio, Vincent JM.
8. *Rape Investigation Handbook* edited by John O Savino, Brent E, Turvey MS, Elsevier.
9. *The Human Skeleton in Forensic Medicine,* 2 edn by Wilton Marion Krogman, Mehmet Yasar Iscan.
10. *Forensic Medicine: Clinical and Pathological Aspects* edited by Jason Pynac James, Anthony Busuthl, Obemomm, 2002.
11. *Human Bone Manual* by Tim D White, Peter A Falkens.
12. *Essentials of Forensic Pathology* by TD Stewart.
13. *Forensic Anthropology* by Steven N Byers, 2008.
14. *Forensic Anthropology and Medicine*, edited by Aurore Schmitt, Eugenia Cunha, Juao Pioheiro, 2006.
15. *Forensic Anthropology* by Peggy Thomas, 2003.
16. *Practical Forensic Medicine,* 2 edn by Francis E Camps, JM Cameron, 1971.
17. *Current Diagnosis and Treatment Emergency Medicine*, 6 edn by C Keth Stone, Roger L Humphries.
18. *Atlas of Human Body: Medicolegal Guide, Medical Jurisprudence* by Samuel Smith, Edwin B. Steen.
19. www.babycentre.co.uk
20. *Human Osteology and Skeletal Radiology: An Atlas and Guide*, Evan Mathes et al, CRC Press.
21. *The Developing Human: Clinically Oriented Embryology*, 8 edn by Keith L Moore, TVN Persand, Elsevier.
22. *Nandy's Handbook of Forensic Medicine and Toxicology* by Apurba Nandy.
23. *JB Mukerjee's Forensic Medicine and Toxicology*, 3 edn.
24. *Parikh's Textbook of Medical Jurisprudence, Forensic Medicine and Toxicology*, 6 edn by CK Parikh.
25. *Forensic Medicine,* 2 edn by PV Guhuaraj.
26. *Medical Jurisprudence and Toxicology,* 7 edn by HWV Cox.

Index